Selected Writings
of Rosemary Ellis

Joyce J. Fitzpatrick, PhD, is the Elizabeth Brooks Ford Professor and Dean of the Frances Payne Bolton School of Nursing, Case Western Reserve University. She is editor of the *Annual Review of Nursing Research* series, now in its fifteenth volume.

Ida M. Martinson, PhD, is the Carl W. and Margaret Davis Walter Visiting Professor of Pediatric Nursing at the Frances Payne Bolton School of Nursing, Case Western Reserve University, as well as Professor in the Department of Family Health Care Nursing at the University of California—San Francisco School of Nursing.

SELECTED WRITINGS OF

Rosemary Ellis

In Search of the Meaning of Nursing Science

Joyce Fitzpatrick, PhD, RN

Ida Martinson, PhD, RN

Editors

SPRINGER PUBLISHING COMPANY

Springer Publishing Company, Inc.
536 Broadway
New York, NY 10012-3955

Cover design by Tom Yabut
Production Editor: Pamela Lankas

96 97 98 99 00 / 5 4 3 2 1

Library of Congress Catalog Card Number: 96-68450

Printed in the United States of America

Portions of this book have previously appeared in the following publications: *Nursing Research*, the *Journal of Nursing Education*, and Springer Publishing's *Annual Review of Nursing Research*, Vol. 1. Permission has been granted for the use of this copyrighted material. The courtesy of the publishers of these publications is gratefully acknowledged.

Chapters 1, 5, 7, 8, 9, 10, and 11 are reproduced with the permission of the family of Dr. Rosemary Ellis.

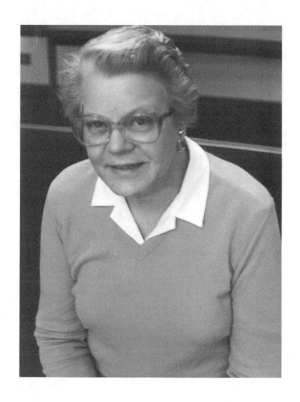

This book is dedicated to the memory of Dr. Rosemary Ellis. The proceeds from the sale of this book will support the Rosemary Ellis Scholar's Retreat at the Frances Payne Bolton School of Nursing, Case Western Reserve University, Cleveland, Ohio.

Contents

Foreword

Dr. Rosemary Ellis was one of the nursing profession's most treasured scholars. She was one of the very first to write on the qualities of being a scientist nurse, of the nature of nursing science, as well as the need for development of nursing theory. Her publications have become classics in the field. Her many awards and honors speak eloquently of her long and very distinguished career. Dr. Ellis was constantly urging attention to the development of nursing knowledge for the improvement of patient care. This book collects many of her previously unpublished writings, as well as some of her classic published works.

Rosemary Ellis was born July 22, 1919. She graduated in 1941 with an A.B. in Economics and in 1944 with a B.S. in Nursing both from the University of California at Berkeley. In 1953 she obtained an M.A. in Nursing Education from the University of Chicago, and in 1964 she received a doctorate in Human Development from the University of Chicago. Clinically, she worked as a head nurse and a supervisor in Medical Nursing at the University of California Hospital and as a Lecturer in the University of California School of Nursing. Administratively, she was the Assistant Superintendent of Nursing at the University of California Hospital in San Francisco, California from 1949 to 1952. From 1953 to 1959, she was an Assistant Professor of Nursing Education at the University of Chicago. During her doctoral studies she was a research assistant in the Department of Psychiatry at the University of Chicago. In 1964, on completion of her doctoral studies, she became an Associate Professor of Nursing at the Frances Payne Bolton School of Nursing at Western Reserve University (now Case Western Reserve University) and an Associate in Nursing at the University Hospitals of Cleveland in Cleveland, Ohio. She was promoted to full Professor of Nursing in 1968 and remained at the Frances Payne Bolton School of Nursing until her death on October 10, 1986.

Dr. Rosemary Ellis had a very special relationship with doctoral students. She saw them as the future of nursing.

Ann Couch of Boston shared openly the experience of being a younger sister to Rosemary. The time spent with Ann was very rewarding as I learned of Rosemary and the key and pivotal role Rosemary played in the family life. Ann shared with me some of Rosemary's memoirs, including letters she had written home from Japan. The detailed description of life in Japan following the war was very moving; Rosemary wrote of her daily life as an army nurse as well as of the people of Japan. Her love for Japan as a country and the Japanese people continued throughout her life.

Dr. Virginia Ohlson, of Chicago, shared her vivid memories of being a faculty member with Rosemary at the University of Chicago and a colleague and friend of Rosemary throughout the years. They were in classes together and rich discussions took place during the years when they were doctoral students at the University of Chicago. In 1968 the two made a trip to Japan together. Dr. Ellis returned to Japan with Dr. Laurie Gunter in 1971 for the first nursing research conference held there. For many years, vacation time for Virginia and Rosemary was spent at Spread Eagle in Northern Wisconsin. Rosemary helped greatly in the care of Virginia's father before he died. Rosemary's first stroke was in 1971 and Virginia Ohlson flew to Cleveland to be with her every weekend for years. They also attended conferences and meetings together. When Rosemary was ill, Virginia came to Cleveland and spent 11 weeks with Rosemary in the last days of her life.

Dr. Rozella Schlotfeldt recruited Dr. Ellis to the Frances Payne Bolton School of Nursing, Case Western Reserve University, when Rosemary was a doctoral student at the University of Chicago. Dr. Ellis's brilliance as a scholar was noted early by Rozella. Dr. Schlotfeldt was most generous with her time, helping me locate various individuals who had knowledge of Rosemary and of her unpublished papers. Dr. Schlotfeldt shared the following handwritten note by Rosemary Ellis in response to Makoto Kikuchi's article entitled "Creativity and Ways of Thinking: the Japanese Style," which was published in *Physics Today*, September 1981, pages 42–51. Rosemary writes:

Enjoyed this very much. I learned from experience that some of my questions make no sense to the Japanese. They do not see the problem that is important to me and I can not express what it is I do not know. Usually over time I come to grasp some better insight but am never ever sure of anything except that I shall never understand fully the Japanese. I do learn from their very different view and ways of operating, however, and that is the source of my fascination and addiction. Pattern recognition of 5000 characters is necessary to "read" Japanese. I know katakana and hiragana the 2 syllable "alphabet" systems, it's the kangi or Chinese characters that are very hard to learn, I know about 250 now. The reasoning behind some of them is fun—confusion or clamor for instance is composed of 3 of the characters for "woman." The character for snow combines rain and sweeping. Snow is rain that can be swept. Japanese working in a committee will get all ideas out and discussed fully and get everybody's feelings and ideas thoroughly out and thoughtfully considered. This takes ages and only at the last minute do they come to an agreement about which option or action to endorse. From then on they together all push to reach the goal. Westerners fairly quickly vote on a goal and general course and spend ages getting clear exactly what they meant or agreed to and getting involvement, commitment and action toward the goal. I think of these different ways of operating often in our faculty actions where lack of understanding and involvement end up in sabotage and inertia.

IDA M. MARTINSON

1

Explanatory Knowledge for Nursing: Forms and Approaches

EDITORS' INTRODUCTION

In the early 1960s, dialogue was beginning among academic nursing leaders about the nature of the discipline. Yet it was not until the early 1970s that this dialogue intensified. Ellis was clearly ahead of her time in presenting these ideas.

Ellis presented this paper as she was completing her doctoral degree from the University of Chicago. She based her arguments on Kaplan's newly published explication of the philosophy of science (1963).

The WICHEN Conferences were annual, regional (Western states), nursing education conferences. Attendees were primarily faculty members from university-based schools of nursing.

Acting and making sense are inherent in human nature and existence. Sensations, and the sense one makes of or from sensations, will direct actions. Sensing, making sense, and acting are not, however, sequential phases or states in a process. They are not linear. They are a

---

"Explanatory Knowledge for Nursing: Forms and Approaches," paper presented at the 19th Annual WICHEN Conference, 1963.

simultaneous and holistic experiencing. The sense made, "explains" or accounts for, the sensation. Sensation is experienced, labeled and accounted for, simultaneously. It is recognized. If it is not experienced, it doesn't exist. If it is experienced, but not identified and accounted for, it perplexes or alarms. The unexplainable is disruptive. Humans are inherently meaning seekers and active. Their activity is not random; it is organized. It is organized by meanings, by created explanations.

Systematized and codified explanatory knowledge is one source of meaning. You can never have my sensations, you can never feel *my* feelings. You can know and use some of my thoughts. *You* can use them, if I am articulate. I use Newton's thoughts, expressed as the law of gravity, to account for falling down and not up, if I stumble. I don't *apply* Newton's law but it explains something. I understand *why* I go down. I account for sensations, I make sense of experiencing. Explanations enable me to act to reduce chances for falling. I have grasped the concept of gravity, learned about it and act on explanation or understanding.

Nursing literature abounds with the phrases "apply theories" or "follow principles." *Apply* and *follow* are wrong verbs. Humans *have* theories or explanations; they inherently create them to account for the state of things or of how and why things happen. Individuals create their own personal explanations or acquire them from others. Children exhaustingly search for answers to why questions. They need to know. Acting and knowing are human essentials.

Effective actions occur with understandings. Nightingale recognized that understanding *whys* was essential for learning how and what to do as a nurse. Theories provide understandings and explanations. Some theories are the formulated, articulated, explicated thoughts of scientists or philosophers that provide explanations nurses use to understand, to act effectively and humanely, and to find meanings. Specification and delivery of care requires explanatory knowledge. Some formulated explanations of others are useful if they have been shown to hold up, to work, to expedite effective actions, or to give comprehensive meaning or understanding of norms such as ethics. At least three approaches to developing explanatory knowledge are essential for nursing philosophy, science, and ethics. The nature of nursing calls for deliberated philosophical stances, explication of values and ethics. Explicated beliefs about the world of humans and human nature. The nature of nursing requires understanding a wide range of myriad facts. Nurses must behave in ethical, humanistic, and effective ways and in a contextual frame of reference that is cohesive and prognostically oriented. Personal idiosyncratic explanations are insufficient. Shared meanings, what we can learn from others, formulated explanations that hold up to test and in use, and knowing who we are, are essential for effective nursing. Explanations accompany and direct actions, and supply meaning, unless we are mindless robots. Debates that pit objectivity vs. subjectivity, induction vs. deduction, empirical or theoretical, humanistic vs. experimental are relatively fruitless and ignorant. Explanations are the goal. Explanations with lasting heuristic power are produced by humans, not methods. Humans sense, feel, and make sense by experiencing and thinking simultaneously. Explanations are the sense that is made by some humans. Reasoning, intuiting, verifying, rechecking, abstracting, communicating, and deliberative discussion of analyzing are human processes that are holistic. Articulated formulations of scientists doing science are spawned in the simultaneity of sensing, feeling, and thinking by the scientist. A nurse's action happens because of simultaneously sensing, feeling, explaining, understanding, and acting.

Kaplan (1963) discusses logic-in-use and reconstructed logic. Logic-in-use is his term for the cognition operating or occurring as one experiences, acts, becomes perplexed, or successfully processes one's world. Such cognition may be deliberative but much of it is not. It includes Polanyi's focal, subsidiary, or tacit awareness and a mix of alogical or illogical thinking. The articulated explanations of scientists, that is, models, theories, laws, or other forms of explanatory generalizations are objectified, idealized reconstructions of the *logic* of logic-in-use. The scientist experiences and objectifies experience. The scientist knows, is objectively aware of knowing and provides explanations and meanings for others to use.

Whether a theory or explanation is formulated from naturalistic observations, participant observations, serendipity, experiments, or reflections on existential encounters, it ultimately depends as much upon the holistic functioning and creativity of the scientist as it does on particular data. The source of formalized explanations, or interpreted meaning of data comes from the sensations, feelings, and idea-tion experienced by the scientist.

But source of objectified formulated explanations is of relatively little importance. What really matters, is whether the explanations are generally useful, whether they "work" or make a significant difference in the doing of others who use them. They are useful if they create meaning for others, meaning that makes a difference. Power to ex-plain, not source or process to formulate is what really matters.

Explanatory knowledge for nursing is necessary to provide under-standing sufficient to create the type of therapeutic structuring that nurses engage in as they strive, by their actions, to produce some delineated beneficence. Explanatory knowledge is required to pro-duce beneficence deliberately. It is also necessary for evaluating the *efficacy* of actions, to know that beneficence *was produced,* and was produced as intended with the least risks or expenditures and fullest benefits.

There are various types of explanations and meanings. Those of interest here are those to be shared with others, or offered to en-lighten. Generalizable explanations of facts are produced by scientists. Comprehensive understandings of particular happenings or of eras are supplied by explanations from analyses and interpretations of historians. History does not repeat but proposed explanations of dy-namics of movements, clashes, development of ideas or technology provides some explanations of antecedents, contextual meanings and developments of significance. History in part explains present status. Recognition and understandings of the roots and consequences of norms and expectations, and comprehensive meaning of meanings are possible from the clarifications and explications of philosophers. Shakespeare's characterizations and plots engage us because they ex-plain recognized repeating patterns in humans and their behaviors. Shakespeare's objectified subjectivities entertain, but they also en-lighten and reaffirm our human-ness. As Kaplan (1963) has observed, our uniqueness as individuals does not mean we share nothing with other humans or that we are not in some ways alike.

Theoretical thinking of nurses, searchings for explanations and for meanings as nurses, has provoked our work to become aware of, and to make explicit, our presuppositions, our explanations, our purposes, our processes, and the phenomena we are concerned about. Nursing models or theoretical formulations present conceptualizations of the goals of the doing called nursing or of the nature of nursing thinking, or of the characterizations of humans appropriate to the purposes, context, and modus operandi of nursing.

Implicitly or explicitly they reveal the types and forms of explanatory knowledge a professional in nursing must have. At the very least these include causal, or functional explanations, moral and humanistic meanings and integrating explanations. Nurses sense, feels, think, and act simultaneously and meaningfully. The sense they make of what they experience directs their actions. Quality and type of explanations used have much to do with effectiveness of their actions.

REFERENCE

Kaplan, A. (1963). *The conduct of inquiry: Methodology for behavioral science.* San Francisco: Chandler Publishing Co.

2

Characteristics of Significant Theories

EDITORS' INTRODUCTION

Ellis's paper, "Characteristics of Significant Theories" was one of six papers presented at a nurse–scientist conference held at the Frances Payne Bolton School of Nursing, Case Western Reserve University, in 1967. This symposium was chaired by Dr. Jeanne S. Berthold. The purpose of the conference was to discuss various positions and approaches to developing a conceptual structure of knowledge useful and necessary to attain the goals established by nurses. The other five papers were; "A Theory of Theories: A Position Paper" by James Dickoff and Patricia James; "Researching Research's Role in Theory Development" also by Dickoff and James; "Theory in Nursing: Borrowed and Unique" by Dorothy Johnson; "A Theory of Clinical Nursing" by Reva Rubin; and "Social Theory in Geriatric Nursing Research" by Myrtle Irene Brown. These are all classic papers, frequently cited as historical documents in the development of nursing science. All of the symposium papers were later published in Nursing Research, *the only research journal in nursing at that time.*

This was a pivotal point in nursing's history. The Nurse Scientist program was developed with federal funding throughout the Division of Nursing. Schools of Nursing were supported to develop doctoral programs in sciences related to nursing (e.g., physiology,

From Ellis, R. (1968). Characteristics of significant theories: Symposium on theory development in nursing. *Nursing Research, 17,* 217–222. Reprinted with permission.

psychology, sociology). Also, individual nurses were provided pre-doctoral fellowships for study at universities where there were nurse–scientist programs. Dr. Ellis, along with Dr. Rozella Schlot-feldt, provided leadership for the nurse–scientist program at Case Western Reserve University.

Theory development relevant to the profession of nursing requires attention to the stated or implied preposition used to connect the word *theory,* or the term *theory development,* to the word *nursing.* The preposition serves to give a sense of placement, direction, or other relationship. Think of the different meanings of the phrases *theories of nursing, theories in nursing,* or *theories for nursing.* It is the intent here to discuss characteristics of theories which are signifi-cant *for* nursing.

The need to attend to the expressed or implied preposition has been mentioned because one is exposed, with increasing frequency, to the term *nursing theory.* This term can be ambiguous. It is used to mean a "generalized theory capable of supporting an overall concept of a process of nursing," as Putnam uses it.[1] In this sense, it means loosely to indicate some, or one, of the concepts used as a basis for explaining or understanding certain nursing practices.

For purposes of the present discussion, the word theory should be understood in its meanings of: "a coherent set of hypothetical, concep-tual, and pragmatic principles forming a general frame of reference for a field of inquiry (as for deducing principles, formulating hypotheses for testing, undertaking actions)," "a systematic analysis, elucidation, or definition of a concept," or "a hypothetical entity or structure explaining or relating an observed set of facts."[2] The task of this paper is to set forth a case for theory development *for* nursing, and to discuss characteristics of significant theories where significant is de-termined with reference to nursing.

The phrase *for nursing* implies that the discussion will be con-cerned only with theories, or characteristics of theories, that are rele-vant to that function which has to do with helping individuals to cope with health problems when their own strength, will, or knowledge is insufficient. Improvement in the practice that achieves this function is the appropriate goal of theory development for nursing. It is this goal which defines the need for theory development, and which, for this writer, determines what is significant theory. It determines what theories, or theories of what, are significant.

Nursing does not occur apart from a patient. This is not to say that all nursing is done in the physical presence of a patient, but that which is nursing is something for or with a patient. It is something that has to do with the patient's response to pathology or the therapy for it, not with the treatment of pathology per se. Nursing also cannot be defined apart from the patient, the definition centers on functions for the patient. Nursing is not defined by the activities of the nurse but by what the patient receives from them. It is not even the process itself; it is the effects of the process.

A significant theory for nursing, therefore, is one that enlightens us about the patient, and what happens to him. With this orientation, studies of nurses may or may not contribute to the development of significant theories for nursing. They have the potential for such a contribution only if they treat the variable nurse as one unit in an interrelationship of units, with patient as an essential one in the structure. Theories which treat the nurse as a determinant in the patient response would seem to have this potential. Theories about why, or what people enter the profession of nursing are far less apt to have this potential.

PURPOSES OF THEORY DEVELOPMENT

Before discussion of the characteristics which make a theory significant for nursing, consider some reasons why nurses need to be concerned with theory development. One elementary purpose for developing theories is to attempt to distinguish fact from pseudofact. Fact is defined as the close agreement of many observations of the same phenomena. By making explicit the phenomena observed, the conditions or context for the observations, and any inferred relationships, one is forced to recognize failure to conceptualize, or observe, potentially relevant variables. If close agreement is not obtained over many observations, either conceptualization is inadequate, or significant variables have not been identified or included.

A second purpose for theory development is that nursing requires the attempt to structure converging facts from a number of fields. This convergence is necessary to the understanding of human beings, especially human beings with health problems. There is no science of human beings. Knowledge about them is drawn from many fields, such as anatomy, physiology, sociology, and psychology. Not one of these fields supplies all the knowledge necessary for the undertaking of nursing human beings. The parts supplied by various fields do not always fit together to make a whole. Nurses and others are far from being able to put forth any grand theories which effectively combine the knowledges about humans already generated from many fields. However, nurses attempt to do this, in effect, in order to nurse. The attempt is essential if one seeks the holistic approach to an individual. Holism, if used as the appropriate view for aiding a patient, requires that one be concerned with any factor, be it physiological, social or any other, which affects the patient's health. It requires that the factors be treated in combination, not in isolation. It also means that the combination is not the same as the sum over each factor. Nursing requires the recognition of the inseparability and interdependence of many factors. Very few concepts or theories from other disciplines effectively enlighten us about the dynamics of interdependent biological and behavioral relationships.

There are theories about illnesses defined as psychosomatic. Rarely do these include propositions to describe, or explain, how psychological factors actually effect the observed physiological changes. What are the mechanisms involved in the translation of a psychological state into biological pathology? The answer is likely to require the synthesis of knowledge across several fields.

Recognition of the interrelationships of biological and psychological factors is the first step toward explaining them and their consequences. For the most part, present knowledge, or theory, is at the level of recognition only. Nursing cannot be achieved through the application of theory or knowledge from several fields unless there is some synthesis. Until formal synthesis is forthcoming, the struggle toward an holistic approach for nursing is held back. Whether synthesis will be produced from the basic sciences remains to be seen. What source will provide a theory of incontinence that will treat all the factors that appear to be involved? Such theory would seem essential for the prevention of the problem, or the treatment or rehabilitation, to the extent possible, of the patient who has this problem.

Another reason for nurses to be concerned with theory development and not merely application, is that theory, or theoretical knowledge, is used to give direction to practice. Only use in practice, and careful observations of results, offer the opportunity for the essential criticism of a theory's usefulness. Practice can and should test theory. Theory cannot be used uncritically. It often is. One can find some examples from nursing where a concept is accepted generally and used without question, where there is very little support for it. One such concept is that of *stages of development.*

There is evidence for a certain order in the progression of development. There is little evidence to support the concept of *stages* in this progression. Stage implies a step-like progression with at least brief plateaus, instead of a slope or gradual continual increase. What evidence is there that stage is the model for the "shape" of development?

Stage is also the term in a model of the course of illness. Stages of illness are believed to exist, but why staging is the model rather than a smooth line of some shape is not clear. That stage may be an inappropriate model here is suggested by the difficulty in defining a stage of illness that is discrete and delimited. Inadequacies of language no doubt contribute. (What is the word to designate a particular point on a curve or a straight line and its position relative to other such points?) But it may make an important difference if individuals are perceived as being in one stage or another where stages are mutually exclusive and in the nature of plateaus, in contrast to being perceived as in some gradual process which is with constant increment and without plateau. Nurses may need to decide which model is most appropriate.

Theory is also useful as a framework for the retrieval and use of generated and stored knowledge which lies in libraries. With a framework there is a guide to knowledges already available but not used, which could produce beneficial innovations. A dentist recently commented that theory development was the most critical current need for development in the treatment of dental caries. According to this dentist, treatment is based on a theory developed decades ago. The theory generally is regarded as inadequate and outdated. Treatment has not changed, however, because no one has come up with a better theory. There is no guide for the direction of change in practice. The dentist also speculated that the separate bits of knowledge to construct a new treatment probably exist in materials already in libraries. It cannot be retrieved and pieced together without some theory as a guide.

CHARACTERISTICS

The above purposes or reasons for nurses' involvement in theory development do not exhaust all possible ones. They are imperative reasons. It is with references to these purposes that characteristics of significant theories for nursing will be discussed.

Scope

Scope is one characteristic important to the significance of a theory. A theory has scope if it covers and relates a number of smaller generalizations or concepts and provides at least a potential framework for ordering observations about a variety of phenomena. The broader the scope, in terms of the number and variety of facts or concepts related, the greater is the significance of the theory. Ideally, theories most important for nursing would be those that encompass both biological and behavioral observations, and have the potential for explaining their relationships. For nursing, the scope should be judged in terms of the generalizations and phenomena pertinent to an individual of the human species in the circumstances which cause him to be labeled by the concept *patient*.

Some of the theories which support current practices lack the scope necessary for nursing. It was long accepted that absolute bed rest was important for proper recovery from major surgery.

Less than 30 years ago many surgeons insisted upon three weeks of bed rest for the patient who had had herniorraphy. Now nurses accept, often unquestioned, the benefits of ambulation in the early recovery from surgery and its concomitants. Both the insistence on absolute bed rest and the insistence on early ambulation stem from conceptualizations based on biological knowledge. There is support for the practice of early ambulation, or maintenance of mobility, in the findings on the effects of stasis, and of the organic changes which accompany immobilization at bed rest over long periods of time. The conceptualizations however, do not all treat all psychological factors which might enter into recovery from surgery. The nonbiological effects of insistence upon early ambulation, and of insistence that the individual resume his care of his body as early as physically possible need to be explored. Biological imperatives may need to be reconciled with psychological ones.

If nursing deals with recovery of the person as well as the body, theory which directs practice must have the scope to cover both. There is need to consider the time and the circumstances necessary for the integration of the *event* of surgery in addition to those which are expeditious for recovery of the body after surgery.

Complexity

Another characteristic of significant theories is that they have complexity; they treat multiple variables or relationships, or the complexity of a single variable. Simple postulations are not particularly valuable if they express only ideas which are readily apparent. There is no objection to the postulation, it simply does not, of itself, stimulate many new insights. If a postulation is of something not obvious, it is most likely complex.

What is complex is often not recognized as such. Incomplete conceptualizations, expressed as simple postulations, are apt to carry the hazards of illusory comprehension. For the scholar, this is unfortunate. For the practitioner who uses the postulation, the consequences may be more severe if he prescribes for others.

Testability

Another characteristic of theories to be used for nursing is that their tentativeness be clearly visible. They should be clearly recognizable as hypothetical. Usefulness of a theory depends upon its being understood as a construct. Constructs are amenable to change. They are frequently changed by their authors. Control over a construct may be lost to the author once it is placed in the public domain. It may not be erased or revised by the public when it should be. The appearance of impermanence of theories is essential if no sufficient scientific evidence accompanies their presentation. The presentation is warranted, but it must be accompanied by the caution that it be used with care and scrutiny.

Testability of theory at a general level, however, is not requisite for use or for significance. It would be desirable. The more useful theories at this time may be those with scope and complexity to the point that they cannot, in toto, be operationalized or scientifically tested in any other way. Testability can be sacrificed in our era in favor of scope, complexity, and clinical usefulness. This is to say that elegance and complexity of structure are to be preferred to precision in the meaning of concepts in the present state of knowledge.

Usefulness

Another prime characteristic, essential for significance of theories for nursing, is that of usefulness for clinical practice. Clinical practice must be the touchstone for determining what theories are significant, and what knowledge nurses must, and should, spend time pursuing.

Theories which may be significant by other criteria are not significant for nursing if they fail in their usefulness for developing or guiding practice. An example of such a theory that may not yet be significant for nursing, but which is deemed significant for other fields, can be found in the construct *dependence.*

Dependence is convenient as a label, but conceptualizations about it are as yet inadequate to the task of guiding nursing practice with adult patients in any important way. Dependence is recognized as a component in illness, it is observed, but what theory guides what the nurse does about it? The global concept dependence includes physical dependence, social dependence, knowledge dependence, or emotional dependence. Theories do not clearly indicate the interrelationships among these. They predominately have to do with a psychological dependence only. Existing theories about dependence expound its genesis. They often contain the implication that independence is the to-be-desired and pursued state. There are many circumstances for which this seems appropriate. The practitioner of nursing, however, deals with dependence as an inevitable accompaniment of whatever calls forth the need for nursing. Theories of the genesis of dependence are not wholly adequate for nursing when an adult suddenly becomes dependent due to illness or accident. Theories with the value of independence are not useful guides for what is to be done about it if it is suddenly or gradually lost forever.

Certainly a goal of nursing is to assist the patient to a state in which he no longer needs the professional. But theory does not give the guidelines for determining the optimum rate to move, or how to treat dependence when prognosis indicates that the patients cannot regain independence.

If our value for independence is prepotent, attempts will be made to have the patient assume full responsibility for himself at the earliest possible moment or to retain responsibility for himself to the last possible moment. Much current practice reflects this. What is often unspecified is responsibility for what. Attempts often are made to move the patient to resumption of independence in management of his physical care without concomittently allowing him resumption of independence for activities or decisions that have to do with his job, home, or other social responsibilities. One could speculate the resumption of independence, or at least abandonment of imposed dependence, for the adult patient, should progress in a rapidly accelerated miniature of earlier life development. Practice would support such theory.

Valuing independence and attempting to maintain it to the last possible moment may, however, be at the expense of learning how to live with dependence. This should be considered when circumstances predict that dependence cannot be avoided, as in chronic debilitating or degenerative disease. Reinforcement of independence by the nurse conveys a high value for it. At what point in time, or in the course of disease which produces erosion of physical independence, does reinforcement of independence hamper acceptance of reality-based dependence? If physical dependence is inevitable, do practices that convey high value for independence increase discomfort with depen-

dence? Do they do the patient unnecessary harm or delay adjustment
to the inevitable? They might make the patient unable or less able to
accept dependence, may make him fear he will be less valued as he
becomes dependent. Stress can be heightened unknowingly if at the
time the patient is becoming dependent, independence is the value
and the expectation the nurse appears to have. The patient's welfare
might be better served if in this case of increasing loss of functioning,
he could learn that he will be accepted and valued when dependent.
This could enable him to retain more easily his sense of worth in the
face of deterioration of his body.

This dilemma for the nurse is the choice between reinforcement of
independence, or creation of an environment in which the patient is
enabled to learn that he can be respected in spite of his physical
dependence, can learn to be comfortable with dependence. Perhaps
the choices are not mutually exclusive, though they seem so. What is
important is that existent theories do not provide help for the practitioner. In this sense they are not yet significant for nursing.

Implicit Values

An implication of the above discussion of dependence is that another
characteristic of significant theories is that implicit values are recognized and made explicit. Theories of behavior usually contain some
implication of the normative or desired behaviors which are not made
explicit. Independence usually is treated as the desired norm or goal
state without reference to the values which cause this to be so, and
without consideration of the values with which it might conflict.

Generate Information

Another characteristic of significant theories is that they are capable
of generating a great deal of new information. Hypotheses which are
highly probable may be so simply because they state what is apparent
empirically and contribute little that is new.[3] A theory that generates
many hypotheses, even some without high probability, or some that
are difficult to test, can contribute significantly to understanding.

Even theories which do not have other characteristics of significance may be significant if they generate hypotheses of some sort.

Hypotheses logically derived, that fail to be supported by empirical evidence, may serve to call attention to variables that were not thought of previously. Variables essential for an effect, or those that can negate effect, may be illuminated, the special case discovered. Incomplete or imperfect theories are better than no theory at all in generating new ideas and new practices. They may be significant. The imperative is to embark on theorizing even at the simplest level, and to cherish the efforts of those who attempt theorizing and the testing of it.

A student's hypothesis about a relationship between stress and helplessness provoked a recognition of the complexity of the concept helplessness. The initial proposition was that feelings of helplessness would be associated with feelings of stress. The study suggested that there is no simple relationship. Under some conditions an individual may feel himself very helpless. If he perceives that he, or the one for whom he is responsible (as in caring for a spouse at home who is in the terminal stages of cancer), is the recipient of adequate help from others, he is not necessarily under high stress with helplessness. He can feel very helpless, but is not threatened by the feeling because others, such as the visiting nurse, help him share and carry out his responsibilities of care. They offer back-up security that, in effect, prevents the feeling that the responsibility is unmanageable. Theory is needed to begin to understand and explore feelings of helplessness and their consequences.

Thinking about helplessness generated recognition of a possible clinical dilemma. Under what conditions should one attempt to offer to act for the person who feels helpless? If one can help him avoid stress by doing for him, should one? Or should the task be to help the individual to gain the competence and confidence to deal with the situation and so to help him attempt to deal with his feelings of helplessness? If the situation provoking his helplessness is self-limiting the dilemma may arise. The nature of a nurse's intervention, what she actually does and the outcomes, are likely to be different for one choice versus the other. Avoidance of stress, and skill in learning what is necessary to overcome helplessness, may not be simultaneously attainable. What theory guides a decision? The gaps in our knowledge and recognition of the inadequacies of existing theories are one result of a very simple hypothesis which itself was stimulated by reading about crisis theories. It could be a significant hypothesis for nursing.

Terminology

A final characteristic of theories significant for nursing would be that they are couched in terminology which can be used meaningfull with, or applied to, phenomena observed in nursing. This might not appear much of a problem, but terminology from one science is used for what appear to be analogous phenomena in another context. The terms, used in this second context, may be expressive, descriptive, and serve as a useful label for the phenomena, but they may have lost their special terminological meaning. The danger is that the loss may not be recognized. An erroneous assumption of analogy is connoted and perpetuated.

Count illustrates the problem in calling attention to the difference between the physical science terms *pressure* and *force*, and these concepts as used in social science.[4] The laws which pertain to pressure and force in physical science cannot be duplicated in meaningful formulas or units of measure in social science.

It is tempting to borrow terminology. An example of one tempting term is "regression in the service of the ego." It appeals as a descriptive label for some of the phenomena observed in illness. An adult defined as ill may be exempted from some responsibilities, is allowed more license for egocentric behavior than when he is well, and for reasons of physical changes, may be fed, bathed, and assisted with toileting. If such a state is functional for recovery, it could readily be called regression in the service of the ego. The phenomenon may not be analogous to those observed by psychologists who use the term to label the conceptualization to "explain" such things as humor, artistic creativity, problem solving, and empathy.[5] Until the analogy is established, use of the term for phenomena in nursing should be avoided even though a more useful label is lacking.

Other terms or phrases attractive for nursing may sound so similar as to be confused in use. *Levels of consciousness* as used in conjunction with anesthesiology or coma is not synonymous with the term *altered states of consciousness* as the psychologist uses it. Unless a nurse who uses them knows the terminologic meaning of phrases from specific fields, they can be confused or used indiscriminately when both psychological and physiological states are involved.

Other Relevant Considerations

Several final thoughts are offered not as characteristics of significant theories for nursing but because they seem relevant. The first is that ultimately, for nursing practice, theories or theoretical formulations will be needed that will predict or explain phenomena for individuals, not groups. Simply knowing that when grouping is based on a cultural factor, that groups differ in their behavior with pain, is not very useful for nursing practice. It does not allow the prediction or presumption that any given individual will behave as the majority of his cultural group appear to behave. It may be claimed that at least the group-based finding could alert the nurse to the probability that a patient from a given cultural group will behave in a certain way. This may or may not be useful. Operating on the prediction is unsafe. It can be biasing and lessen sensitivity to deviations of the individual from specific cultural norms. It may set up expectations which are actually not beneficial for a given patient.

A second thought is that the assumption of the uniqueness of individuals is also not very useful for nursing. When the assumption implies that one knows nothing about an individual until one has encountered and assessed him, it denies the patterning and order in nature. Classification as human begins to tell one something of the structure, basic needs, and of some processes the individual will have. At best, the assumption of uniqueness is useful only as a caveat. It indicates there is risk in prediction and that one must look for individual differences.

SUMMARY

A position has been taken that there is a need for nurses to undertake theory development. Application of theories developed from various sciences cannot be done uncritically. Existing theories, or theories likely to be developed from a single science, are not apt to be complete enough for an holistic view of man. The holistic view seems most suitable for the function of nursing as it is currently defined in the profession of nursing.

Theories that are significant for nursing are those that include the patient as an essential component. They are also those that enlighten us about the patient. Various characteristics of theories, such as scope, complexity, testability, implicit values and others, have been dis- cussed as determinants of significance of theories for nursing. The ultimate test of the significance of a theory for nursing lies in its usefulness for the practice of nursing.

Both methodological development and theory development are es- sential for the inquiry which can facilitate improvement in nursing practice. The domain of nursing practice should delimit the domain appropriate to theory development for nursing. Theory, whether begged, borrowed, derived, or originated by nurses, is significant for nursing if it can enlighten nursing practice.

The first obligation of the professional in nursing is the responsibil- ity for nursing practice or its improvement. This is not to say that contribution to general or specific knowledge is less desirable. It is to say that such concern is less our responsibility than is that for prac- tice. What is significant for nursing, what theory, what knowledge the professional nurse should spend time pursuing, is that which pertains to practice. Generation of knowledge for the sake of knowledge is not the raison d'etre for the profession of nursing—*nursing is*.

REFERENCES

1. Putnam, Phyllis A. Conceptual approach to nursing theory. *Nurs Sci* 3:430–442, Dec. 1965.
2. *Webster's Third New International Dictionary.* Unabridged edition. Springfield, Mass., G. and C. Merriam Co., 1961.
3. Popper, K. Degree of confirmation. *Brit J Phil Sci* 5:146, August 1954.
4. Count, E. W. Dimensions of fact in anthropology. In *Fact and Theory in Social Science,* ed. by E. W. Count and G. T. Bowles. Syracuse, N.Y., Syracuse University Press, 1964, p. 95.
5. Schafer, R. Repression in the service of the ego; the relevance of a psy- choanalytic concept for personality assessment. In *Assessment of Hu- man Motives,* ed. by Gardiner Lindzey and others. New York, Holt, Rine- hart and Winston, 1958, p. 121.

3

Values and Vicissitudes of the Scientist Nurse

EDITORS' INTRODUCTION

The Nursing Research *article, "Values and Visissitudes of the Scientist Nurse" was based on a paper presented by Ellis at the third nurse scientist conference sponsored by the School of Nursing at the University of Colorado on April 3 and 4, 1970.*

As the nurse–scientist programs developed, there was increased national deliberations regarding the nature of nursing science. Ellis's paper highlighted several issues for nurse scientists. At this time there were approximately 2,000 doctorally prepared nurses in the United States, many of whom had their preparation in education. The goal of the Nurse Scientist Program was to increase the supply of doctorally prepared nurses, specifically, those who were prepared as scientists. These scientists were to return to nursing and ultimately to improve the quality and increase the quantity of nursing research. Funding for nursing research in the 1970s was less than $3 million. Ellis's article is still thought-provoking for today's students and scientists. Nursing knowledge still needs to be developed.

From Ellis, R. (1970). Values and vicissitudes—The scientist nurse. *Nursing Research, 19,* 440–445. Reprinted with permission.

Nurses have always known that newborns could see. They acted on this belief, in spite of the fact that authorities told them that newborns could not see. Why didn't some nurse study the question of visual authorities? Why did it wait for the psychologist Robert Frantz to produce the studies that refute the authorities?[1]

There are probably several answers to this question. Until recently, there have been very few nurses with the skill to investigate the question. Secondly, nurses, in the main, have not valued careful, systematic investigation, especially if it should require subjecting newborns or other dependent people to special testing or strange devices. Probably more importantly, the question of whether babies could see or not was not a problem for the nurse. In spite of the words of the authorities, she could act on her own beliefs; she, and the mother and baby, could ignore the authorities' claims, with no consequences. They did not need to pay attention to what scientists said about the infant's vision.

The advent of increasing numbers of scientist nurses should make it more likely that something such as the visual development of infants *would* be studied by nurses. Such scientist nurses, however, will differ from other nurses in the kind, amount, and extent of their formal education. Consequently, they will differ from other nurses in their knowledge, skills, interests, perceptions, and attitudes. Will they differ from the majority of nurses in their values? It seems likely that they will. If scientist nurses are to contribute to the development of nursing, however, there must be some values which scientist nurses and other nurses continue to hold in common. It is to be hoped that one such value would be service to society, expressed as concern and action for health welfare, and the care of the sick.

The route to becoming a scientist nurse, or a career as a scientist nurse, contains experiences and costs which may impede direct expression of this value. Some nurses trained as scientists may even adopt values which supplant the service to society value which underlies nursing. This would not be surprising. A value of knowledge for the sake of knowledge is one that is commonly expressed.

Consider the costs of becoming a nurse scientist through education in some specific discipline. For an appreciable number of years a nurse becoming a scientist usually is removed from daily encounters with a community of nurses, and from living in the environment in which nursing occurs. There is the cost of loss in some nursing skills from disuse, or from the lack of opportunity to keep abreast in a rapidly changing world of nursing practice. There is also the cost in the loss of other learning. While one focuses on learning one discipline, one cannot master others equally important for nursing. The costs affect not only the nurse scientist herself, but may contribute to some estrangement of the nurse scientist from the active nurse practitioner, or to an altered perception of the nurse scientist as a nurse by practicing nurses.

The potential for estrangement is probably related to the motivation underlying a nurse's election of a nurse scientist program or career. Why do nurse scientists choose to bear the costs? The seeking of answers, of knowledge, or status or prestige, of power or influence, of enjoyment, or of special skills are motivation for some. There are probably many more motives, such as avoidance, each with a different potential for producing estrangement from the nurse practitioner.

Whatever the motive for pursuing the career of a nurse scientist, the pursuit is a commitment to a pattern of thought, and of behavior, for years to come. It behooves the nurse scientist to consider how her values relate to those underlying nursing, and to those commonly held by the practitioner in nursing.

The orientation of the nurse scientist to nursing, and to the practice and practitioner in nursing, is essential, if one wants to use the world "nurse" to modify "scientist," or to use the word "nursing" to modify the word "research." Pressures for some discontinuity with nursing can occur in the process of a nurse becoming a scientist.

To truly learn any discipline, one must develop an identity with that discipline. The structures for developing this identity, the spatial or territorial arrangements, and the work relationships, differ somewhat from academic discipline to discipline. Becker and Carper, in an analysis of physiology, engineering, and philosophy found three significant factors in the development of identity with an occupation.[2] These are the informal peer group, the apprenticeship relationship with professors, and the formal academic structure.

In physiology, the vast world of problems yet to be tacked is the perspective. A careful, building block approach through laboratory studies is the mode. Laboratory groups are the vital work and social orientations. The laboratory is the site for peer group interactions. A major professor as a sponsor, a mentor, and perhaps as a life time reference seems the norm. It is not uncommon to find the question "With whom did you study?" to be one of the first questions to be asked of the newcomer physiologist. The answer may influence how the newcomer is perceived or placed. A student typically will select for his investigation some problem specific to the special competence and interest of his mentor. The student will enjoy a close working and social relationship with this mentor which is apt to continue beyond the student's graduation. He spends his time in the same territory as his mentor and does work with or like that of his mentor. He is physically close to the actual working of his fellow students, has frequent opportunity to observe them in action.

The student in a department of philosophy does not have the specific problem focus, the building block rigor, the laboratory work, the laboratory group, or the same sort of professor–student contacts, characteristic of physiology. The professor does his work secluded in his office. The student may consume the completed work, but he rarely can observe the processes, as his professor works on a philosophical problem. Rarely does the student significantly share in these work processes.

Physiology and philosophy probably represent two extreme models, with other disciplines having models more like one or the other, depending on their "hardness" as science.

The process of acquiring identity with and from an academic discipline cannot help but alter the nurse who lives for a significant number of years, as a graduate student, in that academic environment. There may be some tensions during the period if the expected identity with others in an academic discipline fails to mesh with identity as a nurse. Identity as a nurse may impair the perceptions of significant others as they judge the nurse student against the specifications of the discipline identity. The nurse may find some difficulty in accepting the trappings of the academic acolyte, if these are at odds with the nurse identity. Acquiring full identity with the discipline may make one marginal and suspected in nursing. Failure to acquire the identity makes one marginal and suspected in the discipline. How painful is marginality, and what does one do about it? The answers lie in one's values and primary loyalties, which each one must discover for himself. From the disciplines there is the weight of the problems, the ideologies, the fellows, and the sponsors, from that discipline. There is the burden of loyalty to remain what one has become, so as not to let down the sponsor. For a nonnurse disciple, or the nurse whose primary loyalty is to some discipline, this can have important consequences for career opportunities. It can affect the choice of problems or activities one pursues. For the nurse disciple whose nursing orientation remains a primary loyalty, there is greater freedom to the extent that one may move beyond discipleship more rapidly, because there are few masters in nursing. One may lose some security as one moves somewhat away from a discipline sponsor or colleagues, but one can gain a wide freedom of choice of activities, or problems to pursue. Nursing is not currently characterized by sponsorship, or by loyalty to unique or particular ideologies, as essentials in career development.

To be identified with nursing, the nurses need only exhibit a loyalty to the ethos of nursing. Kolthoff, in writing about the nurse scientist, speaks of old traditions of service in new ways.[3] It is clear that to be identified as a nurse one must retain the nursing tradition of service to man, though one can exhibit allegiance to the tradition in a variety of new ways, based on the knowledge and skills acquired in advanced study. Marginality and suspicion can be overcome, it need not be painful, if the nurse scientist has experienced the satisfaction and enrichment that accrues to the professional in nursing, and finds in these the sources for continued willing adherence to the valuable traditions of nursing. In this is a source for renewal through meaningful work. In this is the source for meaningful relationships with practitioners in nursing.

Such sources would dictate that the problems which scientist nurses choose to study, and their perceptions, attitudes, and values, would be those relevant to nursing. They would be those relevant to a special service to man. The nurse, in contrast to some scientists, would ask "Why?" when she starts a search for knowledge, and the answer to why should contain a relevance or reference to nursing.

One should learn from history or the experiences of others. Medicine is today experiencing some dilemma about the orientation and location of its basic sciences or scientists. Some medical school faculty oriented to clinical practice are deeply concerned about the remoteness from clinical skills or problems of the investigations of their colleagues in biophysics or biochemistry. There is a growing schism between some areas of interest of the medical scientist, and the areas of interest to clinical medicine. Seldin illustrates this as follows:

> Successful and important investigations from a biochemical vantage point may lure the clinical investigator in a direction progressively more remote from clinical medicine. The problems posed by patients no longer elicit curiosity. Deranged physiology becomes too complicated for the powerful but restricted tools of basic biochemistry. The net effect may be research not pertinent to any activity in a clinical department.[4]

It is to be hoped that nursing can avoid this pitfall if nurse scientists are primarily oriented to the values of clinical nursing though they need not themselves be engaged in practice.

Some of the vicissitudes of becoming a nurse scientist have been mentioned or can be inferred from the above discussion of values and orientation. Some of these vicissitudes remain in the career of a nurse scientist, and additional ones develop.

There is always the question of "To whom does the nurse scientist relate for communion?" From whom does she seek exchange, stimulation, and a sense of companionship, in the work world? As a member of a very small minority group, the nurse scientist has a rare-zero distribution in the nursing departments of health or illness agencies, and, with few exceptions, in schools of nursing. Nurses caught up in the exigencies of providing nursing care, or of facilitating the learning of beginners in nursing, are not likely to find appreciable amounts of time to give to the nurse scientist, even if they have the inclination or interest. The pace, the locale, and the modus operandi, of the doer and the thinker usually do not coincide. Yet even those who think well alone, or who enjoy the autonomy in research, must, at some point, require the stimulation of response to, validation of, or refutation of, their ideas. For the scientist nurse to achieve this requires that the scientist nurse be willing to become involved to some extent, in the interests, issues, discouragements, and excitements, of the nurse who is not a scientist. Where the values of nursing are evident in the scientist nurse, the gaps between the nonscientist nurse and the scientist nurse are narrowed, to their mutual benefit. The scientist nurse, however, must pick her career arena carefully to ensure that it has the potential for a sense of community in the work world.

The choice of where to work and what to work at, confronts the newly-prepared nurse scientist. Re-entry problems, if one chooses to work in a nursing institution, may plague some nurse scientists. One must become oriented to the institution, to affiliated care agencies, and in some measure, be willing to take on the institution's philosophy and problems. These will be different than those seen as paramount from the graduate student view. There is apt to be a testing by new colleagues of one's identity as a nurse at a time when the new science graduate feels vulnerable or uncertain because of the time-or-distance-from-nursing costs involved in completing a typical doctoral program. Identity challenges recur with any major life transition, and for the nurse scientist, the challenges may come subtly from other nurses.

Then there is the question of "Which language do you speak?" It is amazing to realize how markedly one's language is altered in the process of becoming and being a scientist. Quite unconsciously one begins to use the jargon and special terminology of the world in which one lives. If this is the world of the professional and student in a select discipline, one gradually acquires the language which facilitates communication within the discipline, but does so at the price of impairing communication with those outside the discipline. Even the terms used with some common meaning across sciences, for example the word "variable," if used in communication with the nonscientist, may produce lack of understanding and, possibly, some alienation. Even when one is aware of this hazard, and consciously tries to avoid it, terminology once learned and used creeps into all speech. If one seeks effective communication with nurses, their patients, and their world, one had better use the language of that world, and avoid the terminology of one's scientist training. This requires a continuing conscious attempt to distinguish, and to use appropriately, the languages of two different worlds.

The aforementioned vicissitudes originate from the role of the scientist nurse. What of those in the actual work of the scientist nurse? What of the problems in theoretical study or research relevant to nursing? There are some that arise from the nature of science, and some that arise from the nature of nursing.

First a look at the practice of science. Science is a process for the generation of knowledge. To be useful, the knowledge must be put to some purpose. At times, the scientist's frame of reference may be too narrow for the general good. The development, testing, and introduction of DDT is but one example of some scientist's inadequate frame of reference, a frame of reference inadequate to foresee the important consequences of the use of DDT which are vastly more costly than its benefit. A narrow focus essential to high command of knowledge, techniques, and materials in one sphere, is not the best base from which to consider the universe to which the sphere relates. Analogies to the DDT problem probably could be found in behavioral science practices as well.

Science boundaries are useful for the learner in a scientific community. They limit what he can be expected to master, and give a base for identity of problems. Science boundaries are barriers, rather than benefits, in the *application* of science because of the way they influence the generation and structure of knowledge. Recall the dilemma of medicine. As biochemistry becomes increasingly basic, in the sense of moving to finer and finer particularization, it becomes far less a base for clinical medicine.

A mythical view of science engenders the notion that research finds answers, solves problems, or is an avenue to specific theory. In practice, it is a phase in the vicissitude of theory and research; it is a phase in the alternation of a continuous cycle of theory–research–theory. Far more questions than answers are generated by research. One simply gets another leg up on learning what is yet unknown. In practice, research is more productive for identifying new problems, than it is for giving solutions for empirical problems.

Another view of the practice of science that is open to some question is that significant achievement comes *only* from careful, small, rigorous, sequential studies. Serendipity is recognized as occurring, but no statistics are kept to give insight to the frequency with which chance is an important element in the successful practice of science. What is overlooked in serendipity is the priming of the scientist for a sensitivity for relating heretofore unrelated observations or ideas. Such priming can occur in a variety of ways of which rigorously designed methodical study is only one. Watson's story of *The Double*

Helix is a spectacular example of the triumph of the model builder over the "good guy" methodical scientist.[5]

Objective scientists run the risk of being blinded by theory. Several years before oceanographers paid serious attention to it, a young woman doing routine tasks in the data analysis laboratory of an oceanographer noted a persistent notch in the tracings of soundings of ridges of the ocean floor. She mentioned it to the oceanographer who dismissed it. It did not fit with his theory. Several years later another bit of information caused the oceanographer to recall the notch. With a new frame of reference, the scientist reviewed the tracings of the notch, and a significant breakthrough in the understanding of ocean floor ridges, and a new theory of continent formation and drift, evolved. Now scientists are saying that the continents of South America and Africa were once joined, something the schoolchild of recent generations intuitively guessed from looking at a map, only to be refuted by the scientist of his time. Theory, inadequate facts and limited focus can be hazards for the unwary scientist.

Now for some problems that arise from the nature of nursing. It is said that one knows nothing about something unless one can quantify it. The present capacity of scientist nurses to quantify important variables for the study of nursing is almost nil. The situation is little better even if one elects to study phenomena or variables which are not those of nursing but of something thought to be relevant for nursing. In this era, if scientist nurses limit their research to that which permits measurement, they run the risk of limiting themselves to studying trivia or tangents of nursing. One is forced to premature precision by too stringent a requirement of measurability in the present day in nursing.

Nursing is in an acute state of groping. At best, it has some imprecise labels for many thought-to-be important variables, rather than sound and useful tools for measurement. For some time to come, the scientist nurse must balance the requirements of science with the state of nursing. Too rigorous adherence to the ideals of tight design, careful control, and extensively tested methodologies or tools, can be limiting in this day. Very rarely does clinical research permit such adherence. The hazards in less rigid adherence are to be run, if the scientist nurse seeks to explore clinical problems. Koch in a recent article on psychology, decries scientism because it produces "ameaningful" thinking.[6] (Ameaningful, as defined by Koch, is the world *meaningful* with the prefix *a* where *a* has the same force as it does in words like *amoral*.) Ameaningful thought or inquiry "assumes that inquiring action is so rigidly and fully regulated by *rule* that in its conception of inquiry if often allowed the rules totally to displace their human users," according to Koch. The object of inquiry, in such circumstances, appears to become an "ungainly and annoying irrelevance." Scientism and ameaningful inquiry are as possible in nursing as in psychology.

Some of the problems in inquiry of clinical phenomena can be illustrated from the following examples. Some patients give names to their pathology, or to a body part altered by pathology. A patient with a diagnosis of duodenal ulcer disease spoke of "Mr. Peptic," when he spoke of his ulcer site or ulcer disease. A patient with a crippled hand which was being treated by splinting and physiotherapy called the hand "Monkey." A woman with a colostomy called it "Suzie." A patient with ear noise associated with advancing hearing loss called the ear noise "Cricket."

On the assumption that the naming serves some purpose, it would be useful for the nurse to have some understanding of the phenomena. The case of "Monkey" suggested that the use of the name "Monkey" by the patient and her husband served to achieve some distance and objectivity for the crippled hand. It became a special object upon which special attention, tenderness, and love could be lavished. Each evening the husband would carefully rewrap "Monkey" in its splint. The choice of the name "Monkey" suggests some derision, but it also suggests a pet. It could be seen as an effective coping mechanism for a transitional state.

"Mr. Peptic" was used in another way. As the patient discussed his disease, and his regimens for dealing with it, he indicated that "Mr. Peptic" would remind him if he deviated from his regimens very much. "Mr. Peptic" also would not let him do some things. It appeared as though "Mr. Peptic" was a way of avoiding activities the patient wanted to avoid. "Mr. Peptic" would not let him go to a party if the patient did not wish to attend it.

The naming phenomenon suggests ego alienation. It also provides a short nickname for ease of communication about a diseased body part or process.

From these fragments one can make a case for further study of the phenomenon of patient or patient relative naming of diseased body parts. But how does one study it? One cannot create the phenomenon; one must wait until it comes along. One cannot think of sampling, but what is the population to be studied? How does one study the phenomenon without altering it by the asking of questions? If one simply observes, what does one observe? Piaget's study of his three children on which he bases his theory on the development of reality thinking in the young child offers one method.[7] Even this approach offers no easy solution for the inquiry of the naming phenomenon.

Another example can be drawn from interest in patients' use of humor. This is not something which has been studied, yet it may be another coping mechanism. Some patients seem to use humor as means of transcending a painful experience. This use of humor for transcendence has not been systematically explored. How would one proceed?

Another problem which arises in clinical research in nursing is that of retaining data as the patient moves through time. It is not possible in the present state of knowledge of nursing to anticipate all the possibly important variables. What makes a critical difference is not known. One cannot fully anticipate what should be observed and recorded, therefore one has no entry through a re-run of the data for a variable one has not anticipated. The experiment cannot be repeated with identical subjects. In this time of groping in nursing research, the identification, measurement, collection, and retention of important data, as a patient and nurse move through time, remain problems of great magnitude. Exact repetition of clinical experiments is difficult, because of many patient factors beyond the nurses' control, and it is time-consuming.

Further problems in clinical research can be illustrated from an experience with a widely used personality inventory with a patient sample. In the course of studies of eye surgery, stapedectomy, and general surgery patients, in which the writer has been engaged, the Eysenck Personality Inventory was used to measure capacity for introversion.[8] This variable was thought possibly to be related to having unusual sensory or cognitive experiences under conditions of relative sensory deprivation. One unexpected finding was that the mean scores for various patient groups for the Lie Scale of the Eysenck

Personality Inventory exceeded that of the American norms for the instrument. These norms were, however, based on testing of a college population. The difference might be explainable on the mean age differences between the college sample and the patient samples. It might be due to the fact that because patients with poor vision or eye patching comprised one of our samples, the test had been administered verbally rather than in the written form. The test manual states that the test may be given verbally or in written form, but the norms are presumably based on written administration. Perhaps a higher Lie Scale score results if one is required to respond verbally to questions like "Would you always declare everything at customs even if you knew you could get away with it?" One might be less willing to say out loud, than with a checkmark, that one has a touch of dishonesty. Could the difference be due to the status of patient? All these elements seemed possible. The point of all this is to illustrate that the very limited use of even common psychological tests with a general hospital population does not provide much base for anticipating the outcomes from such testing. There is little base for interpreting test scores from nonpatient norms. Reliable measurement tools developed and used with nonpatient populations may need re-evaluation for use with patient populations.

A final comment on nursing. Nursing is essentially a special type of human caring. Some perceive human caring and science to be antithetical. Science, for some, conjures up images of test tubes, laboratories and increasing remoteness from the real world. This is not the whole story. Science is also the careful measurement of strain in the pinned hip joint, as a patient goes through various movements attendant to selected nursing activities. Measurement of the strain on a hip union during the movement of the patient by means of a draw sheet, or other nursing maneuvers, is for the ultimate purpose of selection or development of nursing maneuvers that produce the least strain on the healing, reconstructed bone. It is a means of achieving a kind of caring that is not simple sentiment, but a kind of caring that includes deliberate, scientifically selected action. Science can be an effective tool of the humanist. It is not his enemy.

Whitehead identified three stages in a process of education: the stage of Romance, the stage of Precision, and the stage of Generalization.[9] The stage of Romance is characterized by the freshness of inexperience. Romance gives way to precision as one learns that there are right ways, accepted rules, and ideologies. Over time, one moves to a stage of generalization. This last stage is characterized by the production of active wisdom. Knowledge is barren until tested and used. Knowledge alone is insufficient, one also needs wisdom. Whitehead states that wisdom comes from freedom in the presence of knowledge. Science and knowledge are the tools of the scientist nurse. Wisdom is an ultimate goal.

The sequential stages of romance, precision, and generalization, characterize the development of the scientist nurse. They also describe a successful nursing career. A young June graduate recently shared the experiences of her first eight months as a staff nurse. She was plunged into responsibilities for which she felt inadequate. Because of the pace and volume of her work, she failed to obtain the satisfactions she had anticipated from nursing. In searching her feelings about nursing, she had come to feel that "nobility is not the thing." Romance had come to an end, as she realized that her romantic view of a Florence Nightingale was not the real world.

Though it is readily understandable why this young nurse feels as she does, one cannot agree with her. From the perspective of more years in nursing, one can see a cycle of romance, to realism, to a return to a sense of nobility that is based on realism. Nobility is the thing in nursing, when "noble" is correctly understood as meaning admirable in dignity of conception, and in manner of expression or execution. There are many ways of expressing or executing nursing. A scientific contribution to the improvement of practice can be a satisfying one for the scientist nurse. It combines the nursing ethos of service to others with great opportunity for self-realization.

This article is based upon a paper presented at the third nurse scientist conference, "Nurse Scientist in Action," sponsored by the School of Nursing at the University of Colorado, April 3 and 4, 1970, and supported by the Division of Nursing of the United States Department of Health, Education, and Welfare, NU 5008-03. Approximately 65 participants from 15 universities attended the conference. Planning committee members were Dr. Betty Jo Hadley, Dr. Margaret Kaufmann, Dr. Rose McKay, Dr. Betty Mitsunaga, Dr. Kathryn Smith, and Dr. Faye Spring.

REFERENCES

1. Fantz, R. L. Pattern vision in newborn infants. *Science* 140:296–297, Apr. 19, 1963.
2. Becker, H. S., and Carper, J. W. Development of identification with a profession. *Amer J. Sociol* 61:289–298, Jan. 1956.
3. Kolthoff, N. Evolution of the nurse scientist; emergence and continued development. *Image* (Sigma Theta Tau) 2:11–12, Nov. 1968.
4. Seldin, D W. Some reflections on the role of basic research and service in clinical departments. *J Clin Invest* 45:976–979, June 1966.
5. Watson, J. D. *The Double Helix.* New York, New American Library, 1969.
6. Koch, Sigmund. Psychology cannot be a coherent science. *Psychol Today* 3:14, 64–68, Sept 1969.
7. Piaget, Jean. *Construction of Reality in the Child,* translated by Margaret Cook. New York, Basic Books, 1954.
8. Eysenck, S. B. G., and Eysenck, H. J. *Manual for the Eysenck Personality Inventory.* San Diego, Calif., Educational and Industrial Testing Service, 1963.
9. Whitehead, A. N. *Aims of Education and Other Essays.* New York, Macmillan Co., 1929.

4

Training for Research

EDITORS' INTRODUCTION

Ellis's article "Training for Research" was published in August of 1970 in the Journal of Nursing Education. *In the 1970s training was an acceptable word to describe the preparation of nurses at the basic level and at the research level. The rigor of research training was evident. Ellis presented a strong argument for nursing to be able to better communicate what it is they do. She gave four logical reasons why doctoral preparation is necessary for nursing. At the time doctoral preparation was not emphasized, there also were only five doctoral programs available in nursing at the time.*

This article has value today as we examine our past to better see our present situation and to think of our future. Dr. Ellis laid a good foundation for advanced education, we need to reread her words.

Nurses are justly proud of their goals, their drive for service to patients, and their general humanistic orientation. There is a remarkable heritage in the traditions of compassion and skilled care in the history of nursing. Nurses have less cause for pride, however, in their ability to communicate what nursing is to others. Noble phrases are readily generated and become the coin for verbal commerce. Recall the

From Ellis, R. (1971). Training for research. *Journal of Nursing Education, 10,* 27–36. Reprinted with permission.

phrase "principles," "comprehensive care," "emotional support," "continuity of care," "nursing interventions," and "nursing science," to name a few. Nurses know what these words mean, to judge by their use, but what do they convey to the public, to physicians, or to other health professionals? When pushed, nurses can convey their *beliefs* and *feelings* about the phrases and their meanings and in some instances can give an example or two to illuminate. But where are the data to support the beliefs, emotions, wishes, and intuitions which underlie the phrases? Do nurses themselves really know, or agree upon, what the noble phrases mean? The time is long past to move from vague generalities, however noble they sound in talking about nursing, if nurses are to be successful in describing and demonstrating the contributions of nursing. With no loss of the humanistic orientation, nurses increasingly will need to attend to matters such as variables, theoretical framework, and outcomes judged by scientific evidence in speaking of nursing practices if they are to be able to speak to others than themselves. The need to improve their ability to communicate outside the profession itself is one reason why research training is an essential for leadership nurses.

An equally compelling reason to require research training in a graduate program in nursing is the need for the improvement of the nursing care of patients. A survey of textbooks in nursing can demonstrate diversity in prescriptions or dictates for nursing procedures and diversity in the rationale or reason given for doing the procedure or practice in a certain way. A recent study[1] highlighted the "contradictory dictates" to be found in nursing texts for positioning the postoperative patient who has had hip arthroplasty. Such contradictions indicate either the total lack, or the inadequacy, of the scientific knowledge used as a base for formulating dictates or guides for practice. Many examples such as this case can be found in nursing literature. Because this is true, nurses have the responsibility to continually strive to improve the scientific base for their practice. It is a professional obligation to those they serve. Nurses must question, study, and constantly seek to improve their practice in the interests of patient welfare. To do this requires that the tools for inquiry and the "rules" for evidence become common knowledge within the profession. Also required is attention to the theoretical frameworks from which orientations to practice derive. Too rarely do nurses recognize or make explicit the beliefs or rationales which guide their practices and appropriately question them.

A third reason to insist that research training is an essential component for the nursing profession is the fact that to date, and for the foreseeable future, nurses will be highly dependent upon basic sciences for the generation of the kind of knowledge nurses require for the skilled nursing care of patients. This makes nurses consumers of science for the practice of nursing, for the administration of nursing, and for the teaching of nursing. If the consumer is not to become a victim of a faulty or biased purveyor of knowledge, he must have at least a beginning knowledge of the nature of scientific inquiry in order to judge the product offered. The hazards in naive acceptance of the outpourings in the behavioral sciences should be obvious. Skipper, Powhatan, and Leonard speak to these in their article on the use and misuse of behavioral science in nursing education.[2] What many nurses fail to take into account is the tentative nature of most of the knowledge in the behavioral sciences. Much of it is still theory to be tested for its empirical validity and usefulness. To be a wise consumer of knowledge in this situation requires some understanding of how knowledge is generated. The state of knowledge in the physical and biological sciences is less tentative, perhaps, than that of present day behavioral sciences, but even here, wise consumption requires insight into how the knowledge was generated and appropriate limitations to its use. Such insight can be increased if one has research training.

A fourth reason can be given to make a case for research training as an essential for the nursing profession. That is the matter of values. Although one often hears the notion that science is value-free, it is a misleading one. Values often dictate what is studied and such things as basic assumptions, contexts, and procedures for work. Generation of knowledge essential to improve nursing practice will need to be done by nurses who are scientists, as well as by non-nurse scientists, if adequate attention is to be addressed to the values thought important in nursing. Values are created or come in to play at all stages of scientific inquiry. They cannot be ignored. Investigators with the values of the nursing profession are needed if significant progress is to be made in the study and the improvement of nursing care.

The need to communicate more clearly and more effectively about nursing, the need to question and improve current practices in nursing, the need to continually function as wise consumers of scientific knowledge generated outside of nursing, and the need to address important nursing values and orientations in scientific inquiry of nursing all require that some nurses become expert in scientific inquiry and theory development. That such expertise is needed is not an issue. Important issues which derive, however, are: What nurses should have such expertise? When should research training be given? What research training should be given?

Should every practitioner of professional nursing receive research training? Desirable as this would be as an ideal, it is clearly not feasible for many reasons. Research training is not acquired in a single course or a single experience. Research requires not only knowledge of the methods of inquiry and of the attitudes of inquiry but also mastery of the content area in which inquiry is made. Such *mastery* is not acquired in introductory or survey courses in the sciences and, for nursing, not in the program appropriately designed to prepare a *beginning* practitioner.

Designers of any curriculum have dilemmas arising from competition among the multiple goals of students and faculties. Perhaps the goals themselves are not in competition, but the time, knowledge, and experiences necessary to achieve multiple goals often produce competition. Most basic baccalaureate nursing curricula are compromises. They have the goal of producing a person ready to begin professional practice. They also often have the goal, expressed or implicit, of enabling the student to move toward self-actualization or some other form of development of self. In some curricula, this includes spiritual development. These goals and that of providing a base for further education are, of course, not incompatible, but the available time and desirable experiences may be. Extended foreign travel to study other cultures could be a very desirable experience, but is not the most efficient way to learn clinical nursing.

The nature of the desirable experiences for full development as a nurse, as a person, and as a life-long learner must be viewed against the need for total numbers and diverse kinds of practitioners, costs in time, money, facilities, and resources, marriage and childrearing goals, and a host of practical considerations. Thus operating curricula for basic nursing programs are compromises. They cannot include all the science each relevant science discipline deems necessary for really understanding and skillfully using knowledge from its field. They cannot contain all the education in the humanities a humanitarian should have. They cannot contain exposure to all the nursing situations a practitioner will encounter.

If they efficiently meet their primary goal of producing persons ready to begin the practice of professional nursing, these curricula are not apt to be able to include all that is essential to produce a scientific investigator or a sophisticated developer of theory. This is not to deny the very occasional exceptional person but rather to claim that a program designed to produce beginning practitioners efficiently is not one that would include a scientific base and research training for all students sufficient to produce the independent investigator or the theoretician. The baccalaureate program should provide an orientation to research and introduce the student to some research findings and their use in relevant science courses and, hopefully, in nursing courses throughout the curriculum, but it should not be designed to produce the investigator or the theoretician. Not every beginning practitioner needs research training to that degree, though honors programs for exceptional students might provide research orientation and some experience beyond that required of every beginning professional practitioner.

When one moves to formal preparation of the master practitioner, however, research training becomes more imperative. The master practitioner, the beginning teacher, or the innovative administrator in nursing needs at least the research training necessary to become an informed, knowledgeable consumer of research. Every graduate of a master's program in nursing should have learning experiences adequate to enable him to become a knowledgeable consumer of research in the sciences basic to his field of practice and of research in nursing. Pertinent learning experiences should include introduction to the philosophy of science, to research design and methodology, and to experiences to augment knowledge from relevant sciences such as physiology, genetics, psychology, anthropology, or sociology, for example. In addition, experiences should include advanced clinical practice based on extended basic science knowledge, theoretical formulations, and scientific observation of patients, their responses, and their problems. All these are fundamental to becoming an informed consumer of research for nursing, but such experiences may be insufficient to produce such a consumer. Experiences in conceptualization, the development of rationale, design, and process, ethics, data gathering, analysis of data, and the production of a scientific report with discussion of findings from systematic inquiry are essential experiences to the production of a knowledgeable consumer of research. The meaning of statistical procedures, of probability, or of design questions, for example, are rarely fully realized unless one has experienced them in one's own idiom, in one's own investigation. Understanding, to the extent that one's thinking is pervaded by an attitude of scientific inquiry and that one uses meanings, not just the techniques, is not achieved by a token experience.

While few will argue with a goal of developing a knowledgeable consumer of research for every graduate of a master's program in nursing, there are many who would not agree that every graduate from a master's program in nursing should design and carry out an independent investigation, to judge from the variance in practices among current master's programs in nursing. This is an issue to be considered by those responsible for conducting graduate programs in nursing.

Nurses cannot hope, realistically, for full colleagueship with physicians or scientists without mastery of attitudes and modes of thinking that go beyond the application of generalizations or formulas or the use of intuition, devices which have characterized nursing practice and the teaching and administration of nursing to date. Nurses cannot hope, realistically, to be key movers in the improvement of patient care or health services without modes of thinking and acting which evidence incorporation of the techniques and values of scientific inquiry. It is difficult to see how such modes of thinking and acting can become inherent without personal experience in every stage of scientific inquiry.

At issue throughout nursing education is how to design programs that will produce the desired experiences for the development of every student to the minimal competence desired as the outcome of that level program. That is, of course, a problem in any professional program anywhere. With in nursing, however, it is an acute problem because each level of program is a terminal one for the majority of graduates, yet it must also prepare some graduates to proceed expeditiously to the next formal level of education. The baccalaureate program in nursing is, and should be, a terminal program for the majority of its graduates, yet it simultaneously must serve as the base for a master's program in nursing. The master's program in nursing is a terminal program for the majority of its graduates, yet it should serve also as the base for entry to the doctoral program. Articulation between bachelor's and the master's programs in nursing could be improved, certainly, but it is not seriously handicapping in the main. The diversity in orientation, content, focus, and goals of master's programs in nursing, however, presents complete lack of articulation or, at best, serious problems in articulation with doctoral programs both in and outside the field of nursing. This is a tremendously significant problem that needs to be solved by nurse educators. Difficulties students face if they consider transfer from one program or school to another cannot be ignored if nursing is to compete for able men and women in our mobile world. Lacks in articulation are general problems in nursing education which cannot be considered further here. They do, however, have some specific consequences when one considers research training. So also are there consequences from the dual function—terminal education or foundation for the next level—of most nursing programs.

A master's program designed for a majority of students for whom it will be a terminal program will likely differ from a master's program designed as an integral step in a doctoral program where the majority of students will proceed through to the completion of the doctoral program. The differences will affect every course or component in the programs, the selection of students, and every other important element of any academic program. At issue then is how to define and design the research training appropriate in graduate education in nursing when, for the present, the master's degree will be the terminal degree for a majority of entrants, and when doctoral programs in nursing are scarce, relatively new, and not oriented to the usual research degree, the doctor of philosophy. What research training should be given to nurses, when should it be give, and by whom remain pressing issues in graduate education for nursing.

Research training involves knowledge and experience in research methodologies and design and command of some definable content areas. It is not enough to simply know something about research design and methodologies. One must also know something about what is under study. It is, unfortunately, all too easy to find examples of research done by nurses (and others) which show inadequacies in knowledge (or at least inadequacies in the use or application of knowledge from the basic sciences), in research design, or in statistics. These deficits can be reduced with more and better formal education courses. What is less easily overcome for nurses is the paucity of role models and mentors who can exemplify expertise in research for nursing for the graduate student.

Although an experience in the conceptualization, design, and actual conduct of an independent investigation is seen by the author as an essential requirement for each graduate of a master's program in nursing toward the goal of development of an informed consumer of research, it is recognized that serious disadvantages could accrue from such a requirement if nurse faculty available to guide students are themselves inadequately prepared for such a responsibility. Using persons who are prepared to guide others in learning to carry out a scientific investigation but who are not nurses presents equally serious problems.

Nurse faculty often lack research experience or expertise. Non-nurse faculty lack adequate experience or expertise in the field of nursing. In both situations the student and the profession of nursing suffers. If a school of nursing offering graduate programs lacks sufficient numbers of nurses adequately prepared to serve as faculty and to guide the research training of students, but acknowledges the disadvantages of turning over the guidance of nurses to non-nurses, that graduate faculty in nursing must search its collective soul to decide which disadvantage it must inflict on graduate students. The choices—omission of the minimally desirable investigative experience or an experience with inadequately prepared mentors or with mentors with insufficient working knowledge of nursing—are not pleasant ones for any nursing faculty. The profession owes it to its young to remedy the situation. Omission of an investigative experience in the programs which produce the majority of nurse faculty at present, the master's program, can only perpetuate current inadequacies in the preparation of nurses for faculty roles.

It is the author's observation that students in graduate programs in nursing have some disadvantages that graduate students in other fields of study may not have. These disadvantages arise from the following facts. First, there is a lack of coherent theories of and for nursing which are widely discussed and taught and which provide a framework for development of empirical research. Learning theories, personality theories, cognitive development theories, and the like can serve to stimulate identification of researchable problems for students in psychology, for example. There is no analogous pool of theories for nursing practice for the student of nursing to draw upon. Secondly, it is common for the graduate student in many fields to become immersed in research attitudes, procedures, and strategies through an apprentice-type association with faculty involved in research. The problem pursued by a student investigator is often based upon, extended from, or tangential to ongoing research of his faculty. While this has the potential disadvantage that what the student chooses to study may be limited to what his faculty is willing to spend time on in view of their own interests, it does serve as a natural and comfortable introduction to research and researchable problems for many students. It is also a vehicle for student–faculty associations in common work which can have many rewarding and lasting consequences for both. The typical student in a graduate program in nursing has no chance for such opportunities and associations. Nurse faculty, in the main, are not engaged in work in which the graduate student can have a rewarding colleagueship. This situation is regrettable for student and faculty alike. It makes identifying a worthwhile, feasible area for investigation that much more difficult for the graduate student in nursing. Finally, a third disadvantage is that the instruments and methodologies used in many studies by nurses are of necessity borrowed. For example, psychological tests not specifically designed for nursing situations may be used in the interest of using tested, reliable instruments. But they may represent approximations of the variables in which nurses are interested at best or lack testing in the clinical population of interest to a nurse. If one does not find a useful approximation in a ready-made test, the process of instrument development or assessment is added to the steps in inquiry. This is no small problem. Finding or developing instruments or learning various technologies such as those borrowed from physiology, for example, frequently add to the tooling-up time for a graduate student in nursing who embarks on an empirical investigation. These are not just problems for individual students; they are problems for the profession of nursing.

Development of a scientific attitude and mode of thinking does not come simply from inclusion of an investigative experience in a graduate program. It develops only if all the courses or experiences in the curriculum convey this attitude and mode of thinking. The mode of thinking is as desirable in clinical nursing as it is for the generation of knowledge. Clinical courses, and clinical practice experiences in these courses, should reflect an orientation to inquiry. A master practitioner of nursing, a teacher of nursing, or an administrator ought to draw upon knowledge that is available knowing the *limitations* of the knowledge. He learns this skill in courses in clinical nursing, courses in methods of teaching or evaluation, or courses in organizational science as well as in courses whose content is philosophy of science or research design and methodology. The interrelatedness of all parts of a successful curriculum—and thus the need to change all courses in the curriculum if one changes a major component or adds a major component such as "development of a scientific attitude"—is a basic tenet in Malone and Berkowitz's discussion of the development of research skills in graduate nursing students.[3] How many graduate programs in nursing reflect such cohesiveness of attitude throughout all courses? One would expect it to be a rarity if one views the lack of cohesiveness everywhere else in nursing. One cannot expect cohesiveness within curricula, across courses, unless there is cohesiveness in faculty attitude and practice. Without inhibiting opportunity for sound, carefully designed experimentation, those involved in graduate education in nursing need to agree upon generally acceptable expectations of the clinical competencies, the research skills, and the teaching and administrative skills minimally essential for the master's graduate. Failure to agree on these expectations can only prolong the present state of chaos for the public, for potential entrants to graduate programs, and for the graduates and their employers.

If a master's program is the appropriate level for development of the skills essential for knowledgeable consumption of research, one must look to doctoral programs to produce those capable of becoming independent investigators, theoreticians, and sophisticated critics of research. An introduction to critique of research is a desirable experience for the baccalaureate and the master's program student. However, it is this writer's view that the knowledge and skill required to become an independent investigator and to critique research in any depth cannot be obtained in the time reasonably allocated to the primary purposes of either the baccalaureate or master's preparation in nursing. But what kind of a doctoral program can prepare the nurse for a career as an independent investigator or theoretician?

Very few schools of nursing today have sufficient well-prepared faculty to consider offering a doctoral program in nursing whose primary purpose would be development of nurses for the role of career investigator in nursing. The distribution of schools of nursing with research programs of such stature that they could begin to offer potential arenas for the education of nurses for the role of independent investigator is that of rare to zero. The organization of content in nursing, of knowledge in the state of theory to be tested or of knowledge deriving from limited research, is also seriously deficient as a base for a doctoral program aimed at producing investigators. This should be an issue for those in graduate education in nursing specifically and for the profession generally.

Individual nurses have sought research training beyond that appropriate at the master's level through study in scientific disciplines. This is a long route for many nurses and has the disadvantage of being indirect. The problems of interest to scholars in basic science disciplines are almost all tangential to nursing if they are relevant at all. A given problem of interest to sociologists may have some components which would be of extreme interest to nurses. However, the orientation of the sociologist qua sociologist must differ from that of a nurse qua nurse. Sociology and nursing may share interest in given phenomena, but they do not share a common orientation or raison d'être. They do not share identical goals. Learning research skills and orientation through sociology, through study of sociologic problems, or through any other discipline is better than no or inadequate research training. It is not the ideal way imaginable to learn to become a sophisticated investigator of nursing phenomena. With inadequacies in the field and in the resources in nursing today and the disadvantages of training outside nursing, how should nurse educators proceed in advising nurses who seek research training? How should nurse educators proceed to remedy the inadequacies for such opportunities

within the field of nursing? What must be done at present to increase the pool of nurses who can become career investigators or
theoreticians in nursing and who can create the climate, organize
the knowledge, and function as role models for future generations of
nurse investigators. Current solutions will have to differ from desirable future solutions given current inadequacies in schools of nursing.

For the foreseeable future, all available avenues for the attainment
of skills for investigation and theory development must be used by
nurses who seek a career as investigator or teacher. These avenues
presently are study in the basic sciences and study in programs lo-
cated in schools of nursing. The profession and its educators need to
foster further development of sound doctoral programs in nursing.
Research-oriented programs leading to the Ph.D. should augment programs that are strongly oriented toward clinical nursing or nursing
education.

The bias of the writer for inclusion of an independent investigation
experience in the master's program should be apparent, and it ex-
tends also to the doctoral program. This position is taken in full recognition that in other fields there is considerable concern about the
dissertation requirement and criticism of the length and research
emphasis of Ph.D. programs.[4] Such concern evidences the need to
consider the advantages and disadvantages of a program leading to a
professional degree and the advantages and disadvantages of a research-oriented program leading to the research degree. There is no
question but that both are needed for the nursing profession.

Graduate programs in nursing should offer students an opportunity
to become informed and critical consumers of research. Few would
rationally argue that an ability to use research reports intelligently is
not required for a teacher of professional nursing, for the administrator of a nursing service, or for a master practitioner in nursing. Development of this ability should be a minimal expectation of every student who graduates from a master's program in nursing. Failure to
ensure this is to handicap the graduate for the roles he is apt to be
expected to fulfill. There is great need, also, to augment the all too
scarce supply of nurses capable of significant investigation and theory
development for nursing. These are the challenges of today for graduate education for nurses.

REFERENCES

1. Lygre, Laurae: Loads on the Femoral Head during Nursing Activities after Internal Fixation of the Hip by Means of a Radio Telemeterized Nail-Plate, unpublished master's thesis, Case Western Reserve University, 1970.
2. Skipper, J. K., J. W. Powhatan, and R. C. Leonard: "The Use and Misuse of Behavioral Science in Nursing Education," *Journal of Nursing Education,* 8:23–26, January, 1969.
3. Malone, M. F., and N. H. Berkowitz: "Development of Research Skills in Graduate Nursing Students," *Journal of Nursing Education,* 3:5–7, 37–42, August 1964.
4. Miller, J. P.: "The Master of Philosophy: A New Degree Is Born," *Journal of Higher Education,* 37:377–381, October 1966.

5

Humans as Instruments of Science

EDITORS' INTRODUCTION

The decade of the 1970s was a time when doctoral education in nursing advanced beyond the nurse–scientist phase to programs based in Schools of Nursing, with the degree offered either a DNSc or PhD in Nursing. The PhD program in nursing at Case Western Reserve University began in Fall 1972. By 1981, Ellis had made a full recovery from her stroke (suffered in 1972) and was teaching the required doctoral level nursing theory courses. Her contributions to nursing knowledge development peaked in the early to mid-1980s.

Knowledge can be acquired in many ways. The type of knowledge correctly labeled science is that generated and validated through processes that are communicable to others and subject to review and critique in the light and heat of accepted expectations and norms of peer scientists. The processes for development of knowledge of a scientific nature are those of theory construction and research in dynamic interaction.

As nurses increasingly value research, seek a validated body of knowledge for nursing purposes, and engage in the scholarly pursuits for which universities exist, research and research methods have gained attention with emphasis, it seems, on methods or "how to do

"Humans as Instruments of Science," written September 9, 1981.

49

it" to the neglect of sufficient delineation of the important knowledge questions to be addressed by whatever methods are appropriate to the questions and the phenomena to be studied.

It is a premise of this paper that the nature of the question and the phenomena to be studied mandate methods for study rather than that method is the determinant. It is also a thesis of this paper that the generation of knowledge involves discovery and validation and the processes for these are related but distinguishable phases and differ considerably. Few would argue this but it is common among those who functionally seem to equate research and science to focus only on the testing and validation processes. This is natural because discovery as a process is not reducible to one ordered set of procedures to be followed or some algorithm. Discovery is individualistic; it can be serendipitous; it is a function of mind-set, interest, opportunity, personality, happenstance, and creativity. Stories of great discoveries or insights recounted by their originators describe the uneven, idiosyncratic processes in discovery and the beginnings of what, if science is produced, is a long process of formulation, formal formulation and testing, reformulation and testing. Total development from wonder to insight, to testable question to scientific knowledge moves from one individual mind to increasingly impersonal, public, objectifiable, systemized, validated knowledge of a distinctive type called science.

Undue or premature emphasis on particular formal research methods may neglect the very early discoveries antecedent to formal theory construction. Such discoveries are essential and are individualistic and creative. Preoccupation with formal methods seems to occur in nursing at the expense of discourse on the nature of the important questions to be addressed in a nursing knowledge system. Dominant nursing perspectives today, extant nursing models or metaparadigms vary, but all include humans as a critical element along with other highly abstract complexities. To produce science from such abstractions in the deep chasm between these mind-made abstractions and general ideas and sense data perceivable through some direct or indirect observations must be recognized and overcome in some way. The ability to share, to review, to communicate in a common language, to argue the correspondence between ideas and data are necessary to produce science. Theoretical structures of science must have some tie or potential to be tied to observables, to be subject to research processes, to be claimed as scientific.

If one accepts that all models to portray the idea *nursing* require the concept *humans,* then one perforce must consider what knowledge about humans is required in a nursing knowledge system and what observable realities of humans could provide the data for the scientific portion of that knowledge system.

If human responses, human perceptions, human experiences, and human capacities for both alteration and constancy characterize something of the nature of knowledge that might be essential nursing knowledge, then what are the methods to discover and validate such knowledge? Certainly scientist nurses must know the general methods of science and be able to learn and utilize specific methods in use in different sciences as appropriate to the phenomena, goals, theoretical structures and questions focal to a particular field if the scientist nurse's question is of that sort. But a nursing perspective often is not identical with that of another science, and an adequate nursing knowledge system will not be generated solely from knowledge bits and pieces from other sciences, nor will such sciences formulate nursing questions.

All this is to say that scientific knowledge is that which is publicly verifiable; it is generated by communicable processes and consists of facts and interpretations of facts organized in some mind made conceptual structures which link observables to produce meanings and frames for operations and understandings. If understandings sought are understandings of human actions and responses in health of illness, then what are appropriate instruments for systematically studying human actions, responses, and meanings of the class or categories necessary for nursing knowledge? Certainly humans themselves can be such instruments. Who but another human can experience and report what a particular human behavior evokes or is apt to evoke in other humans, or hypothesize about the function of a particular behavior? Who but humans can recognize, try to understand and communicate the appearances and feelings labeled sadness? Who but humans can experience human sensations, attempt to describe them verbally, by analogy, or in some innocuous way as a possibly helpful source for mitigation of aversive reactions to unavoidable unpleasant, frightening, or not yet experienced stimuli?

Kaplan's (1964) exposition of *act meaning* and *action meaning* is a useful discussion for consideration of study of human behaviors with a goal of scientific knowledge. A kind of understanding of humans that comes from within by means of empathy, intuition, or imagination could be one source in the discovery phase of knowledge generation along with knowledge from without that grows from systematic careful observation. Field work and naturalistic observations are other strategies in which the human investigator is the most effective tool for initial insights and conducting the dynamic interplays of wondering, hunching, formulating, checking, and reformulating that typically precede formal postulating and subsequent rigorous testing, replication, and acceptance.

Science as product comes from processes that are known, reproducible, with necessary controls, and the product is integrated in or produces reformulation of some conceptual structure. Science as process contains some phases in which the investigator as human is a particularly effective instrument. Piaget's ability to study and ponder the discrepancies he inferred between an infant's schema and adult concepts and thinking produced his heuristic description of how the sensory–motor phase of infants' and young childrens' learning eventuates in the separation of self and work object and awareness of the permanence of objects. His formulations could then be tested, critiqued, or studied by others. The initial observations and insights were not dictated by research method, and undue concern with particular methods could be restrictive or counter productive to the creativity of the heuristic scientist in development of theory to be tested.

Premature preoccupation with formal process may be handicapping to the development of a nursing knowledge system if indeed knowledge of some particular class of human perceptions and misperceptions, human feelings, human sensations, and human responses are among the realities that nurses observe and attempt to understand in a nursing context. Impersonality is essential in the testing of theory or a hypothesis; it may inhibit effective use of one's self in the initial insights essential to systematic development of adequate knowledge of the human phenomena of interest to nurses as nurses.

REFERENCES

Kaplan (1964). *The conduct of inquiry.* New York: Chandler Publishing Co.
Margenau (1973). The method of science and the meaning of reality. *Main Current in Modern Thought, 29*(5), 163–171.

6

Philosophic Inquiry

EDITORS' INTRODUCTION

Ellis believed that the potential contribution of philosophy to nursing knowledge development had been recognized, however, it has not been realized. She was at the forefront of critical thinking that is essential for all scientists in the development of knowledge. She continued to urge nurse scientists to search for the roots of their inquiring and to ask questions about the logic, clarity, and significance of the research questions in nursing.

Science in nursing had expanded greatly in the decade from 1973 to 1983, as evidenced by the growth of doctoral programs in nursing, the increase in federal research funding targeted for nursing, and the number of nurses prepared at the doctoral level. The Annual Review of Nursing Research (ARNR) *series was initiated through the leadership of Harriet Werley, founding editor, who believed that the science had matured significantly, and that there was enough research in key areas to support the review series. Ellis's review of philosophic inquiry in nursing was commissioned as one of the first chapters in the first volume of the series. Ellis also was invited to join the first Advisory board of the ARNR series.*

From Ellis, R. (1983). Philosophic inquiry. In H. H. Werley & J. J. Fitzpatrick (eds.), *Annual review of nursing research* (vol. 1, pp. 211–228). New York: Springer Publishing Co. Reprinted with permission.

Nursing research predominantly has developed through the use of research and theory construction processes in empirical science. Much of the knowledge needed for professional nursing practice is of the nature of empirical science. There are other ways of knowing, however, other realms of meaning that are also important in nursing. Philosophy is one of these realms. It is another important way of knowing.

The knowledge base for nursing practice includes empirical science, but it also must include clarification of values, ethics, and study of the nature of knowledge or ways of knowing essential to professional nursing practice. A few nurses have engaged in philosophic inquiry in the quest for nursing knowledge. The *potential* contribution of philosophy to nursing knowledge development has been recognized. As yet it has not been realized.

Silva (1977) wrote of the need to examine the role of philosophy in deriving nursing knowledge. She identified three implications for nursing research pertaining to the inherent interrelatedness of science, theory, and philosophy. The following statements quoted from Silva present her thesis.

1. Ultimately all nursing theory and research is derived from or leads to philosophy.
2. Philosophical introspection and intuition are legitimate methods of scientific inquiry.
3. Nursing knowledge arrived at by the scientific method too often sacrifices meaningfulness for rigor. (pp. 61–62)

Silva addressed the relationships among philosophy, theory, and science. She also exposed the limitations for nursing of overemphasis on scientific method and rigor before a philosophical stance is established and significant nursing questions are identified and considered. Current activity in model building and grand theories of nursing practice are searchings for meanings and philosophic stance.

Beckstrand (1978) identified logic and ethics, both of which are branches of philosophy, as components of nursing knowledge and later (1980) noted that "many aspects of philosophy are entailed in the knowledge used in nursing" (p. 78). Carper (1975/1976), in her philosophic inquiry, identified ethics as one of four fundamental patterns of knowing that are found in nursing literature. Her own inquiry demonstrated the contribution, not limited to ethics, that philosophical investigators can make in nursing. A report of a part of the Carper investigation has been published (Carper, 1978).

The need for philosophic inquiry arises not simply from the need for logic and ethics or from the need for study of the nature of knowledge, but also from philosophic questions called forth by the fundamental nature of nursing. Such questions as the following must always be considered by nurses. What does it mean to be human? What is the meaning of dignity? What does it mean to be compassionate, humane, and caring? What is nursing? Such questions cannot be answered from the data or facts of science. They cannot be studied by impersonal, objective experimentation. The questions are sweeping, broad in scope, and value-laden; they defy final answers. They are questions professional nurses cannot ignore. Philosophic inquiry is the avenue by which nurses can address such questions.

Philosophic inquiry is inquiry to extract or clarify meanings from existing knowledge. It is used to make manifest and to clarify values; to identify ethics; and to study the nature of knowledge. Scientific research is a search for new formulations. It arises from the need for new knowledge and inadequacies in knowledge. It is done for some purpose that is tied to the perspective and beliefs of the investigator. Philosophic inquiry is used to expose, clarify, and articulate the perspectives, beliefs, conceptualizations, and methods that characterize a field. Through philosophic inquiry, scholars attempt to make known the good or desirable and the effective means to such ends. Philosophic inquiry makes explicit perspectives, methods, and the norms for the acceptable.

However one chooses to answer the philosophical question of what is nursing, it is apparent that the goals of nursing are the health and welfare of humans. These goals, as Curtin (1979) pointed out, are not scientific; they are moral. They are a seeking of good. They call for philosophic inquiry to clarify means and ends.

In attempting to articulate goals and modes for attaining goals, nurses have philosophized about nursing. Philosophies of nursing have been written for over a century. Many present-day theories or models are more philosophies of nursing or philosophic perspectives than theories or models from science. Most of these theories or models have not been developed or communicated in the method of philosophy. The theories or models have been attempts to articulate the essence of nursing, to identify desired goals, the good. Their authors showed their beliefs about the nature of human beings, human potential, and nursing. The models are individual statements of the oughts of nursing; they are projections of the desirable. They convey beliefs and stances toward some purpose. They are products of wisdom, experience, intuition, introspection, and values. They are not products of scientific or formal philosophic inquiry. They are sometimes called philosophies of nursing in the common usage "philosophy" but not in the usage of "philosophy" as a discipline.

Philosophy as a discipline is concerned with eternal problems such as the relation between mind and body or the nature of knowledge (Rorty, 1979). Philosophers endeavor to see reality as a whole. They analyze the nature and findings of different branches of knowledge; they examine the assumptions on which they rest and the problems to which they give rise. Philosophers seek to establish a coherent view of the whole domain of experience (Kneller, 1978).

Phenix (1964), in his system for the logical classification of realms of meaning, identified philosophy as a synoptic field, comprehensive in scope.

> It is concerned with every kind of human experience and not with any one domain. . . . All dimensions of all kinds of experiences come within its purview. . . . The distinctive function of philosophy is the interpretation of meaning. . . . *The meanings expressed in philosophy are meanings of meanings. . . .*
>
> The method of philosophy is essential that of dialectic, a process of conceptual examination, examination by raising questions, proposing answers, and developing implications of those answers in continuing cycles. . . . In philosophic inquiry the question is more important than the answer, for the answer, if accepted as beyond question, stops inquiry. [Phenix, P. H. *Realms of Meaning.* New York: McGraw-Hill, 1964, pp. 253, 254. Used with permission.]

Philosophy seeks explication of meanings, not measurement of concepts. It provides logical semantic, and conceptual analyses, not formulations or reformulations to organize facts or to generate new theories. It is argumentative, directed at examination of presuppositions and implications, and at the determination of what logical relations do or do not obtain (Flew, 1979).

Carper (1975/1976), in her philosophic study of ten years (1964 to 1974) of nursing textbooks and journals, noted the shift in nursing language from observational to conceptual. Conceptualizations, conceptual analyses of various sorts, concern for ethics and values, and for essential meanings are now common in nursing literature. More formal philosophic inquiry is clearly appropriate and essential in nursing. The purpose of this chapter is to review the philosophic research that has been done by nurses from the first study by Newton in 1949 to February 1982.

The usually identified branches of philosophy are epistemology, that branch that investigates the origin, nature, methods, and limits of human knowledge; metaphysics; logic; and ethics. These branches did not prove useful for organizing a review of nursing research. No studies of nursing or by nurses were found to be in the branches of metaphysics or logic. Only the Carper (1975/1976) study could be considered as epistemology, and only two studies, those of Sternberg (1979) and Norberg, Norberg, and Bexell (1980) dealt with ethics. Philosophic studies done by nurses were studies of nursing using the methods of philosophy. They are useful for nursing. They are not classifiable by any single branch of philosophy. They also cannot be classified by any formal taxonomy for nursing research that exists.

In the absence of an established system for organization of the comprehensive field covered by philosophic inquiries in nursing, organization, for purposes of this review, was created by four general areas in which nurses were found to have made formal inquiry as philosophers. The review will be presented under general headings for the four areas; (a) ethics; (b) philosophy of nursing education; (c) concepts, values, and processes; and (d) methodology. These areas are not necessarily mutually exclusive. Some studies touched upon more than one area. The areas do serve to group studies and present a general picture of nursing research that stems from philosophy.

ETHICS

General societal concerns for ethics and the implications of developments in science and technology have resulted in growing attention to
ethics in general, to bioethics or biomedical ethics, to ethical issues in
human rights and human experimentation, and to professional ethics.

Investigations pertinent to ethics are beginning to appear in the
nursing literature. Applegate (1981), Davis (1981), Ketefian, (1981a,
1981b), and Murphy, (1976/1977) are empirical studies of nurses or
students in nursing. These studies were not philosophical inquiries
and are not reviewed here. The Mooney (1980) study of ethical components in four nursing theories also was not a formal philosophic
inquiry. Only two studies in this area were found that qualify as formal
philosophic inquiry, those of Sternberg (1979) and Norberg, Norberg,
and Bexell (1980).

Sternberg (1979) undertook a search for a conceptual framework
as a philosophic base for nursing ethics. Sternberg defined ethics as
the philosophy concerned with morality, its problems and judge-
ments. Ethics is concerned with how one uses morality in life situations, with the oughtness, obligations, and rights in life. Sternberg
identified and analyzed four concepts that might serve as a philosophic foundation for nursing ethics. Each of the four is now used, or
their meanings exist, in nursing practice. They are different philosoph-
ically and have disparate connotations and implications. The four
concepts are *code*, the present instrument utilized by the profession
to promulgate ethical standards; *contract* (not defined by Sternberg);
context, where the arena in which ethical conflict occurs is the determinant of ethical response; and *covenant,* a formalized agreement
between persons to do or not to do something specific. Sternberg did
not make clear how contract and covenant differ. The presentation of
the concepts and discussion of their implications are highly informa-
tive. They would be useful to all nurses concerned with defining or
delineating nursing ethics. They could also be useful to those who
teach ethics in the context of nursing.

Swedish investigators Norberg, Norberg, and Bexell (1980) used
both empirical and philosophical inquiry to study ethical problems
arising in the feeding of patients with advanced dementia. The condi-

tion of patients with advanced dementia may deteriorate to a point where spoon feeding is no longer possible or safe. The alternative of forced feeding by intubation has its own evils and dangers. Starvation is unacceptable. This real and common ethical dilemma for nurses involved in the care of patients with extremely advanced dementia provoked the study.

Norberg, Norberg, and Bexell (1980) made careful observations over a four-week period on wards where long-term geriatric patients were provided care. During these observations, the investigators held repeated discussion with the nurses caring for the patients. The observations and discussions provided material for philosophic analysis. From this analysis, five conflicting demands that created ethical dilemmas for nurses were identified. The consequences of the dilemmas and avenues for resolution were explored. The report of the study was too brief and lacked the detailed discussion of the conflicting demands of dilemmas necessary for a substantive contribution to nursing knowledge. The investigators were concerned with calling attention to the existence of dilemmas and to the need for further study of them. There was insufficient detail and explication in the report. It did, however, provide one model for beginning philosophic inquiry of nursing ethics.

There is a great need for continued systematic inquiry from many approaches to the study of ethics, ethical dilemmas, conflicting demands that defy resolution, and nursing ethics as conceived and lived by nurses. Philosophic inquiry has been used very little in the vital area of nursing ethics. Such inquiry is greatly needed. Philosophic inquiry has been used to a greater extent, and for a longer period of time, in research on nursing education.

PHILOSOPHY OF NURSING EDUCATION

The earliest identified philosophic inquiry done by a nurse was that of Newton (1949). It was an investigation of the philosophy of nursing education of Florence Nightingale. The study was based on interpretation of Nightingale's concepts of reality, man, God, religion, standards, means and ends, goals, education, and nursing education. Nightingale's beliefs were then related by Newton to three schools of philosophical thought—scholasticism, idealism, and pragmatism. The conclusion Newton drew was that Nightingale was eclectic and quite pragmatic. The investigation provided insight into the philosophic tenets basic to Nightingale's activities and prescriptions. The prescriptions have had a lasting impact on American nursing. Newton's contribution has been to identify their philosophic source. Whether the prescriptions are valid for contemporary nursing depends upon the usefulness of pragmatics as a major mode for decisions and whether the pragmatically based prescriptions from the 19th century are still valid.

Nightingale was also a focus for Barritt's (1971/1972) investigation. Barritt analyzed Nightingale's writings to study the values that could be identified regarding nursing education. Barritt used the headings for the National League for Nursing criteria for appraisal of baccalaureate and higher degree programs in nursing as a taxonomy for the study. The Nightingale values and those of contemporary baccalaureate education in nursing were highly correlated, according to Barritt.

History and philosophy overlap when history of ideas or values are at issue. The Barritt study is not primarily concept clarification; it is more a study of premises and oughts. It is a demonstration of continuity over time in nursing. Schuyler's (1975/1976) study of Nightingale and Louise Schuyler used history and philosophy to delineate the philosophies of nursing education of these two nurses. Their philosophies of nursing education were presented in the context of their era and their general philosophies of life. Schuyler the investigator also related the two nurses' views to reigning philosophies of education of their times. Schuyler's inquiry added little to further understanding of Nightingale beyond that provided by Newton (1949) or Barritt (1971/1972). There are other historical figures in American nursing that warrant study besides Louise Schuyler. The study does not have general usefulness for nursing.

Philosophical inquiry of nursing education that coupled such inquiry with empirical study also was found. Both philosophic inquiry and an empirical study were done by Vaillot (1926) on commitment to nursing. From an existential viewpoint, Vaillot sought to resolve the opposition or separation between the Habenstein and Christ (1955) classifications of nurses as traditionalizers and utilizers. Vaillot rejected the either/or classification. She identified commitment as the critical element in nursing. She characterized nursing education as a passage from existence to being. Vaillot's analysis of the Habenstein and Christ concepts of traditionalizer and utilizer was dialectic. Synthesis was accomplished with the concept of commitment. Commitment became the essential good for Vaillot. Vaillot also did an empirical study of the worlds of students in nursing. She asked students in collegiate, diploma, and practical schools of nursing to answer with whom they identified and what their appraisal of nursing as a profession was. For Vaillot, education for commitment to nursing was the essential and ultimate good for nursing education. Commitment was identified as crucial for authentic being as a nurse. The means to this end was not explicated. It is not at all clear why the empirical study was done or how it contributed to the advancement of Vaillot's thesis or to nursing knowledge.

Commitment, along with *caring* and *presence,* were identified by Nelson (1977/1978) in a philosophical inquiry of ideas in nursing literature that corresponded to ideas of the existentialist philosophers Martin Buber and Gabriel Marcel. The intersubjectivity in the nurse–patient encounter was identified. Commitment was viewed as necessary for selfhood in nursing. This view is identical to that of Vaillot. Commitment was also deemed by both Vaillot and Nelson to be vital to the future of the nursing profession.

Caring was viewed as essential to self-actualization of the nurse. Nelson also thought it was essential for rendering care in the interests of the other. Presence, or being there subjectively, was also considered to be essential for care. Presence, however, created a potential for difficulty in that it requires self-disclosure and availability. Nelson's discussion raised questions that beg answers through philosophic study. Are there limits to commitment, caring, or presence? How much is it reasonable to expect a nurse, as nurse, to open up to a patient or client? Is there such a thing as a professional relationship? Is it different from other human relationships? If so, what are the differences? What are the implications? What are realistic expectations? What are the norms? What are the limits? Inquiry in this area has not yet been done; it should be done.

CONCEPTS, VALUES, AND PROCESSES

A Greek nurse explained the Greek derivation of the word "philosophy" (Lanara, 1976). The word literally means "love of wisdom." Lanara viewed philosophy as helping one to develop a coherent world view, one that makes sense of everyday experience. This world view was described as an outlook; a body of values; and a synthesis of spiritual, moral, humanitarian, and social values by Lanara.

The heading *Philosophy, Nursing* in the *International Nursing Index* is used for listing articles on nursing theory, personal or institutional philosophies of nursing, concepts, and much else. The increase in the number of listings under the heading is quite striking since the first volume of the index appeared in 1966. The increase attests to more conceptual analyses and to concern for meanings in nursing. Part of the search for meanings is through philosophic analysis of concepts, discovery or extraction of concepts from literature, and search for values.

Six investigations of concepts, values, or meanings that qualify as philosophic research were found. The six investigations are only similar in that they are philosophic inquiries and were done by nurses. The six investigators have begun work that must be done to make manifest a nursing perspective or world view, if one indeed does exist.

The first study in this group is a study of empathy by Zderad (1968). As a philosopher, Zderad inquired into the nature of empathy, its ingredients, and processes. She also delineated the synthesis process by which her construct, empathy, was developed. The description of the synthesis process is a contribution to nursing methodology. It was Zderad's logical contention that nursing requires both the objective view, as found in science, and the subjective view. The subjective view as thought to be essential for knowing in the intersubjectivity of the nurse–patient relationship. Subjectivity, as evident in phenomenology, also was considered valuable because of the very nature of nursing practice. Nursing practice is concerned with both objective and subjective realities of the human beings involved—nurses and patients. Empathy, for Zderad, requires subjectivity. It is lived.

Phenomenology is a philosophy and a method of inquiry. The method is used to describe and understand events or other phenomena as they are experienced and lived. Subjective meanings and intuition are used to understand the experiencing as lived. Phenomenology can be used to elucidate the experience of illness as lived, for example. Nurses must seek to understand human responses to illness, if they are to nurse effectively. Phenomenology may contribute to the understanding. It was Zderad's thesis that empathy cannot be understood or studied solely from objective scientific processes. Empathy may be a learned skill; it is also a philosophic stance expressed through art in nursing. Synthesis of objectivity and subjectivity occurs in the nursing act. There is synthesis of several realities and synthesis of art, science, and experience. Knowledge development for nursing practice must explore methods for synthesis. The Zderad study is a contribution in this area. It is an example of the process of synthesis.

Health and its various meanings were the objects of Smith's (1981) investigation. The study was a critical analysis of the foundations of various meanings of health. Smith sought to explicate, clarify, and extend knowledge by logic and reasoning and presented four different ideas of health that she found in the literature. She tested them by the method of testing ideas in philosophic inquiry, that of critical discussion. The four models of health identified by Smith were:

1. eudaimonistic—health as a general well-being and self-actualization;
2. adaptive—health as a condition of capability for effective interaction with the physical and the social environment;
3. role performance—health as measured by effective role performance; and
4. clinical—health as the absence of morbid physical or mental condition.

Smith argued that nurses need to think of health from the adaptive or eudaimonistic orientation and thereby to become guardians of the quality of life in the community.

Accepting this function for nurses appeals as a laudable ideal, but it would be difficult to realize. Realistically, there is a myriad of variables that affect the condition of existence of any individual or group. It is totally unrealistic to expect nurses to be responsible for, to be able to treat, or to manage all the variables of existence. Although it is impossible to define operationally or to evaluate quality of life, this should not rule out an argument for rejection of the clinical model of health for nursing. Smith's critical discussion of the four models provided nurses with a clearer view of the differences and the range of models of health. It did not explain how the models could be used. Further work is needed to show how the elucidation of the models can lead to further development of nursing knowledge or practice. The Smith study did provide a useful approximation for the beginning of order in the ambiguous meanings of the term "health."

Healing was the focus of Homberg's (1980) inquiry, in which roots of healing were identified in the Bible. Homberg concluded that the biblical tradition of the healing power of respect for human worth and dignity, of interpersonal relationships, of community, and of meal fellowship have parallels in contemporary nursing. The significance of this conclusion is unclear. The observed parallels to biblical tradition are not unique to nursing. It is reasonable to expect some biblical influence on nursing, given the centuries of involvement of religious communities in nursing. The study does indicate some conditions for, or components of, healing. This is useful for nursing.

A value may be a subject for philosophic inquiry. Raya (1975) characterized the nursing profession as a treasury of values. What these values are and how they are manifest has not been delineated or investigated. Only one study, of one nursing value, was found for this review. It is that of an investigation of heroism as a value (Lanara, 1974). (This doctoral dissertation also was published as a book in both Greek an English; see Lanara, 1981.) With the purpose of enriching and redefining nursing philosophy, Lanara (1974) examined the concepts and images of heroism as they related to nursing. Philosophy, including primary sources from classical Greece and the Byzantine period, and philosophic nursing literature was used. In addition, writings of Nightingale and statements on nursing from the International Council of Nursing, the World Health Organization, and nursing leaders were analyzed. The values of responsibility, respect for human dignity, and sacrifice were illustrated in relation to the concept heroism. The concept heroism was deemed relevant to nursing situations. The heroism of love for fellow human beings in need of care was an idea Lanara (1974) found to permeate nursing philosophy. Nursing philosophy was viewed by Lanara (1976) as a reservoir of values that can provide criteria for choices nurses must make for the benefit of the served other and the living spirit of care. Lanara's concept of heroism, which encompasses respect for human dignity, is somewhat different from the common American concept of heroism. The element of sacrifice elucidated by Lanara (1974) raises for nurses questions similar to those identified earlier in this review about commitment. Commitment and sacrifice have been expectations in nursing. The extent to which they are current expectations remains to be studied. Meanings, norms, and limits must also be investigated.

Meaning in suffering, treated as a nursing dilemma, was the subject of another investigation. Kreidler (1978/1979) used an existential and spiritual framework to articulate an approach intended to humanize the nurse's encounter with those who suffer. The approach was offered as an alternative to the need for self-control and control of others to protect against feelings of helplessness. In the investigation, the terms *spiritual, existential,* and *suffering* were clarified from contemporary literature in philosophy. Nursing literature on spirituality and existential themes also was examined. A conceptualization of human beings as spiritual persons needing to find meaning in life and in suffering was explicated. Transcendence was considered a desirable potential that might be realized, depending upon how one viewed and used suffering. A nurse's personal philosophy was thought by Kreidler (1978/1979) to be important for facing the suffering of others. It was also thought to be important for its consequences in nurse–patient interactions. The Kreidler study should be valuable for nurses involved in care of patients with cancer or other long term or catastrophic health problems. It may also be of more general use for understanding nursing. It could help nurses recognize or formulate their personal philosophies. It could help in understanding or patterning behavior.

The sixth study in the group was a study of a process, in contrast to a construct or value. The subject of the study was judgment. Doona (1975) sought to clarify the judgment process in nursing. She contributed a theory of judgement to systematized nursing knowledge (Doona, 1976). Doona (1975) reviewed and critically analyzed the implied or stated views of judgment of major philosophers. She identified two pivotal thinkers, Saint Thomas Aquinas and John Dewey. The theories of judgment of these philosophers were synthesized by

Doona to form a new theory. Phases of judgment and varieties of judgment such as common sense, speculative, and pragmatic, were considered in the context of nursing. Doona's (1975) theory of judgment was delineated in a paradigm and operationally defined. The study's consequences for improvement in decision making in nursing practice could be considerable. Doona (1976) demonstrates the practical utility that may accrue from philosophic inquiry.

METHODOLOGY AND NURSING

Methodology is a branch of logic dealing with principles of procedure. Principles of procedure specify how knowledge is produced and the criteria for its acceptance as knowledge. Methodology is the study, description, explanation, and justification of methods. Five philosophic studies by nurses were found. They can be grouped by their common focus on methodology and nursing. In other respects they are quite dissimilar. They are reviewed in chronological order.

The first study, by Paterson (1971), proposed a method for nursing research developed from synthesis, application, and conceptualization of philosophic ideas in relation to Paterson's beliefs about what she terms "professional clinical nursing." Paterson identified her study as methodological inquiry directed at understanding the process, rather than the products, of scientific inquiry. "Nursology" was Paterson's term to designate the study of nursing aimed at the development of nursing theory. Paterson's method of nursology was presented in a five-phase model. The model was a description of a subjective–objective method of study Paterson thought was essential for, and specific to, the humanistic nature of nursing. Concern for the humanistic traditions of nursing is pervasive in nursing literature. Many nurses think the emphasis on science and on the generality and objectivity that characterize science threaten nursing practice traditions. For some, scientific objectivity vitiates or violates the humanitarian essence of nursing. Polarization of science and humanitarianism seems to be occurring. Philosophers strive to provide the synoptic view. Paterson's inquiry is an example of the synthesis that must be achieved in the development of nursing knowledge. If such knowledge is to serve as the base for practice, science and humanitarianism must be synthesized. Paterson's inquiry offers one model for the process of synthesis. There must be continued study of the process of synthesis. There is need for a synoptic view of what are treated as disparate areas of knowing in nursing. As manifest in nursing practice, these disparate areas must create a whole.

Another study to clarify the process for theory development in nursing was that of Walker (1971a). In Walker's inquiry and in an article based upon it (Walker, 1971b), nursing was considered in the context of discipline. Discipline, defined as a community of scholars who share a common orientation to a domain of inquiry, and to the principles for the production of knowledge, is not generally understood in nursing. The Walker (1971a) inquiry in the context of discipline demonstrated the difference between knowledge-development procedures and principles and the nature of nursing as a practice. Nursing practice has as goals the health and welfare of human beings. Nursing, as practiced, is a humanistic resource for health. Knowledge-development procedures serve as means for extending knowledge. They are independent of the uses of knowledge or a practice.

Whether nursing is or should become a discipline remains to be explored. There is some evidence of communality in thinking in nursing as noted by Donaldson and Crowley (1978). However, as Donaldson and Crowley pointed out, there is no single method of inquiry in nursing. Science, history, and philosophy are methods of inquiry that seem essential in nursing. What is the structure for a body of knowledge that is produced by such distinctive approaches? What synthetic processes are required to create a meaningful whole? The substantive and methodological structures for a nursing discipline need to be explicated and the work of Donaldson and Crowley (1978) and of Walker (1971a) and Carper (1975/1976) continued.

Traditional science as a threat to nursing values was evident in the Taddy (1975/1976) investigation. Taddy noted that examination of the historical development, the assumptions, the concepts, the prejudices, and the methods of traditional science imperil the preservation of the unique and personal character of human beings. Taddy found evidence in nursing literature of resistance to the potential loss, through generalization, of the human aspects of persons. She felt that nurses, as scientists, must reconcile objectivity and generality with being humane, with subjectivity, and with individualism. Knowledge about humans generated from objective and subjective studies is essential knowledge for effective nursing practice. What Taddy identified as at issue is: What views of humans are appropriate, for what purpose, and for what questions? These are questions nurse investigators must consider and investigate as philosophers. The pervading traditions of nursing would seem to require preservation of all that the concept person has connoted in nursing. Exactly what it does connote or what it is intended to connote remain unstudied areas for which philosophic inquiry is a useful method of investigation. Other methods of inquiry should be examined to ascertain their usefulness and compatibility with nursing views of human beings.

A brief treatise on nursing and methodology was found in a letter to the editor of *Nursing Research*. The contribution of the author (Zbilut, 1978) warrants mention in this review. Zbilut noted that there were epistemologic constraints to the development of a theory of nursing. Zbilut claimed that viable methods depended upon social decision for validation, that it is not possible to create viable models or to assume perspectives incongruent with envisioned practice. Models of envisioned practice must submit to the test of social decision for viability. Zbilut identified four "habits of thinking" (p. 128) in viewing human nature. These are:

1. empiriological—experiential (scientific research and personal experience),
2. empirical—metaphenomenal (hypothesis, theory, law),
3. philosophical—metaphenomenal (human contingencies of man's existence viewed with regard to a space-time axis), and
4. philosophical–transcendental (formalities which embrace being with precision from the space-time axis).

According to Zbilut, participation is the only way some things can be known. Knowing another person as a fellow human being, for example, cannot be achieved from objectivity and mere observation. Zbilut's position endorses phenomenology and indicates limits of the empirical–metaphenomenal habit of thinking for producing a theory of nursing. It is useful to have Zbilut's brief identification of the four habits of thinking. All four have been used to seek nursing knowledge.

The four habits encompass the approaches advocated by Donaldson and Crowley (1978). The taxonomy accommodates Paterson's (1971) nursology. What remains to be developed is a methodology of nursing for the integration of the various views of human nature resulting from the different habits of thinking. There is also need to ponder the habit of thinking that can produce the socially congruent viable model of nursing.

The investigations and considerations of methodology have raised questions about the particular nature of nursing practice. They have raised questions about the knowledge base essential and sufficient for that practice. How nurses think, their values as a collective, their reflections, and what counts as good must be studied further through philosophic inquiry and discourse. At present, a case has been made for scientific, philosophic and historical research in nursing. Emphasis has been on scientific research. The usefulness of the generalizations that are the products of science seems not to be questioned. What has been overlooked, except by philosophers in nursing, is the continuing need for knowing the particular that is required by the nature of the human responsibilities entailed in effective nursing care. What is also to be sought is the wholeness in knowing. A search for nursing meanings, begun with Zderad's (1968) study of empathy, Lanara's (1974) study of heroism, and Kreidler's (1978/1979) study of suffering must be continued and expanded. There is also a need to confront complex, comprehensive questions. There is need to examine, for example, what it means to be compassionate, humane, and caring toward patients. There is need to explicate the nursing meaning of person, or the meaning of "being there," or the meaning of dignity. Philosophic inquiry is required for these tasks.

SUMMARY

Criteria for the evaluation of philosophic inquiry in nursing are logic, clarity, and the significance of the questions or problems for nursing. An additional criterion might be the meaningfulness of the inquiry for enlightenment and for ordering understandings and meanings in nursing. On all of these criteria, the relatively few philosophic inquiries by nurses are generally acceptable and make a contribution to nursing research. They begin to explicate and clarify meanings from existing knowledge. There are very few nurses who have become philosophers. It is essential that this pool be enlarged. Continuing inquiry is needed to examine and explicate other meanings, to further methodology for nursing knowledge, and to identify and explicate nursing values and ethics. The domain of human experience in illness must be explored further to provide knowledge vital for nursing practice. Practice requires a synthesis of the various ways of knowing. This synthesis must be manifest in the ways of being, in doing for and with another person.

Too many of the studies reviewed here were doctoral dissertations that did not result in publication. The reasons for this are not known. Perhaps it is part of a more general picture of the fate of a proportion of dissertations. It could be, however, that review panels and editors of journals are not familiar with philosophic inquiry or that the purposes for which a journal exists are too narrow to accommodate reports of philosophic inquiry. It was abundantly clear to the reviewer that indexing systems in nursing are not very useful for cataloguing the comprehensive scope of philosophic inquiries. The indexing systems reflect the absence of a comprehensive, coherent taxonomy for nursing research. The problem is a general one for nursing research. It is particularly acute for research that is philosophic.

Finally, it is easy to differentiate science, history, and philosophy in the abstract. Ultimately, in the human experience of knowing, they must become a whole. By and large, philosophy has been neglected by nurses, or it has been considered only superficially. The neglect and superficiality are a detriment to nursing and nursing-knowledge development. The potential of philosophic inquiry for nursing is largely unrealized.

REFERENCES

Applegate, M. I. Moral decisions in selected clinical nursing practice situations (Doctoral dissertation, Columbia University Teachers College, 1981). *Dissertation Abstracts International,* 1981, *42,* 1818B. (University Microfilms No. 81–22, 930)

Barritt, E. R. B. Florence Nightingale's values regarding nursing education (Doctoral dissertation, Ohio State University, 1971). *Dissertation Abstracts International,* 1972, *32,* 4029B. (University Microfilms No. 72–4418)

Beckstrand, J. The notion of a practice theory and the relationship of scientific and ethical knowledge to practice. *Research in Nursing and Health,* 1978, *1,* 131–136.

Beckstrand, J. A critique of several conceptions of practice theory. *Research in Nursing and Health,* 1980, *3,* 69–79.

Carper, B. Fundamental patterns of knowing in nursing (Doctoral dissertation, Columbia University Teachers College, 1975). *Dissertation Abstracts International,* 1976, *36,* 4941B. (University Microfilms No. 76–7772)

Carper, B. Fundamental patterns of knowing in nursing. *Advances in Nursing Science,* 1978, *1*(1), 13–23.

Curtin, L. L. The nurse as advocate: A philosophical foundation for nursing. *Advances in Nursing Science,* 1979, *1*(3), 1–10.

Davis, A. Ethical dilemmas in nursing: A survey. *Western Journal of Nursing Research,* 1981, *3,* 397–400.

Donaldson, S. K., & Crowley, D. M. The discipline of nursing. *Nursing Outlook,* 1978, *26,* 113–120.

Doona, M. E. A philosophical study of judgment for use in nursing. (Doctoral dissertation, Boston University, 1975). *Dissertation Abstracts International,* 1975, *36,* 1369A. (University Microfilms No. 75–20, 918)

Doona, M. E. The judgment process in nursing. *Image,* 1976, *8,* 27–29.

Flew, A. Preface. In J. Speake (Ed.), *A dictionary of philosophy.* New York: St. Martin's, 1979.

Habenstein, R. N., & Christ, E. A. *Professionalizer, traditionalizer and utilizer.* Columbia: University of Missouri Press, 1955.

Homberg, M. A. Biblical roots of healing (Doctoral dissertation, Columbia University Teachers College, 1980). *Dissertation Abstracts International,* 1980, *41,* 1310B. (University Microfilms No. 80–22, 117)

Ketefian, S. Critical thinking, educational preparation and development of moral judgment among selected groups of practicing nurses. *Nursing Research,* 1981, *30,* 98–103. (a)

Ketefian, S. Moral reasoning and moral behavior among selected groups of practicing nurses. *Nursing Research,* 1981, *3,* 171–176. (b)

Kneller, G. F. *Science as a human endeavor.* New York: Columbia University Press, 1978.

Kreidler, M. C. Meaning in suffering: A nursing dilemma (Doctoral dissertation, Columbia University Teachers College, 1978). *Dissertation Ab-*

stracts International, 1979, *39,* 4813B. (University Microfilms No. 79–09001)

Lanara, V. A. Heroism as a nursing value (Doctoral dissertation, Columbia University, 1974). *Dissertation Abstracts International,* 1974, *35,* 2848B. (University Microfilms No. 74–26, 597)

Lanara, V. A. Philosophy of nursing and current nursing problems. *International Nursing Review,* 1976, *23,* 48–54.

Lanara, V. A. *Heroism as a missing value.* Athens, Greece: Publications Sisterhood Eviniki, 1981.

Mooney, M. M. The ethical component of nursing theory: An analysis of ethical components in four nursing theories. *Image,* 1980, *12,* 7–9.

Murphy, C. P. Levels of moral reasoning in a selected group of nursing practitioners (Doctoral dissertation, Columbia University Teachers College, 1976). *Dissertation Abstracts International,* 1977, *38,* 593B. (University Microfilms No. 77–16, 684)

Nelson, Sr. M. J. The thoughts of Martin Buber and Gabriel Marcel: Implications for existential encounters in nursing (Doctoral dissertation, Columbia University Teachers College, 1977). *Dissertation Abstracts International,* 1978, *39,* 222B. (University Microfilms No. 78–21, 826)

Newton, M. E. *Florence Nightingale's philosophy of life and education.* Unpublished doctoral dissertation, Stanford University, 1949.

Norberg, A., Norberg, B., & Bexell, G. Ethical problems in feeding patients with advanced dementia. *British Medical Journal,* 1980, *281,* 847–848.

Paterson, J. S. From a philosophy of clinical nursing to a method of nursology. *Nursing Research,* 1971, *20,* 143–146.

Phenix, P. H. *Realms of meaning.* New York: McGraw-Hill, 1964.

Raya, A. C. Psychiatric nursing: A conceptual approach. A textbook for Greece (Doctoral dissertation, Columbia University, 1975). *Dissertation Abstracts International,* 1975, *36,* 1149B–1150B. (University Microfilms No. 75–20, 233)

Rorty, R. *Philosophy and the mirror of nature.* Princeton: Princeton University Press, 1979.

Schuyler, C. B. Molders of modern nursing: Florence Nightingale and Louise Schuyler (Doctoral dissertation, Columbia University Teachers College, 1975) *Dissertation Abstracts International,* 1976, *37,* 1179B. (University Microfilms No. 76–20, 875)

Silva, M. C. Philosophy, science, theory: Interrelationships and implications for nursing research. *Image,* 1977, *9,* 59–63.

Smith, J. A. The idea of health: A philosophical inquiry. *Advances in Nursing Science,* 1981, *3*(3), 43–50.

Sternberg, M. J. The search for a conceptual framework as a philosophical basis for nursing ethics: An examination of code, contract, context and covenant. *Military Medicine,* 1979, *144,* 9–22.

Taddy, Sr. J. A philosophical inquiry into existential philosophy as an approach for nursing (Doctoral dissertation, University of Pittsburgh, 1975). *Dissertation Abstracts International,* 1976, *36,* 1369B. (University Microfilms No. 76–14, 173)

Vaillot, Sr. M. C. *Commitment to nursing: A philosophic investigation.* Philadelphia: Lippincott, 1962.

Walker, L. O. Nursing as a discipline (Doctoral dissertation, Indiana University, 1971). *Dissertation Abstracts International,* 1971, *32,* 3459B: (University Microfilms No. 72–1528) (a)

Walker, L. O. Toward a clearer understanding of the concept of nursing theory. *Nursing Research,* 1971, *20,* 428–435. (b)

Zbilut, J. P. Epistemologic constraints to the development of a theory of nursing. *Nursing Research,* 1978, *27,* 128–129.

Zberad, L. T. A concept of empathy (Doctoral dissertation, Georgetown University, 1968). *Dissertation Abstracts International,* 1968, *29,* 936A–937A. (University Microfilms No. 68–12, 814)

7

Knowledge for Nursing Practice

EDITORS' INTRODUCTION

Although it is not certain what specific audience Ellis wrote this paper for, the paper included an important theme for Ellis, that is, the need to evaluate not only the generation of knowledge, but also its transmission and utilization. Ellis continued to stress the relationships between research and practice (utilization of knowledge) and research and education (transmission of knowledge). In this paper, as in many of her other writings, Ellis draws upon her own experience with illness and recovery in discussing nursing science development.

Nursing research can only be understood or advanced within the context of a dynamic whole called nursing. Nursing, taken as a whole, is oriented simultaneously to three endeavors with regard to knowledge. First, nursing has to do with the transmission of knowledge. This takes place in educational programs that have as their goal the preparation of practitioners, educators, administrators or researchers in nursing. The process of education, or the transmission of knowledge

"Knowledge for Nursing Practice," written February 27, 1984.

occurs through organized and directed learnings. The transmission of knowledge involves goals and processes somewhat different from the goals and processes of nursing practice or nursing research. You are all familiar with the goals and processes of education, so let me move to consideration of nursing practice and nursing research by consideration of processes, goals, and knowledge.

Nursing practice is a central part of my nursing whole. It is concerned with the utilization of knowledge. It required the utilization of knowledge in a deliberate and artful way to produce the goal of beneficence for which nursing exists.

Nursing research, the third element in a meaningful nursing whole, is the development or advancement of knowledge for nursing. All three processes, the transmission of knowledge, the utilization of knowledge, and the development of knowledge, are the obligations of professionals.

The transmission of knowledge has been an object of study in nursing for years. As a process it is not controversial and can be related to practice with little difficulty. We are less clear about the relationships between the development of knowledge and utilization of knowledge in practice.

From reviewing the research and theory development literature in nursing for the past 20 years, it is apparent that the relationship between practice and research, or between practice and theory has been and remains a controversial issue. Wald and Leonard, Conant, and many others have argued that nursing practice should dictate nursing research. Their position is that nursing practice should be the source for nursing research questions, and nursing practice should be the site for nursing research.

An opposite view has also been supported. This opposing view is held by those who do not wish to be limited by nursing practice as it is. They have visions and aspirations for what practice could and should become. These nurses see nursing research as shaping, changing, and improving nursing practice. Obviously, both sides are right; we need both points of view. More importantly, we need to think of nursing as a whole. We must create systems that facilitate a free flow of ideas, problems, concerns, values, and knowledge, between and among practitioners, educators, administrators, and investigators. All of us must be concerned about knowledge for nursing.

Let me consider nursing practice and nursing research from a focus on knowledge and particular types of knowledge. Nursing was called an art and a science by Florence Nightingale. The term "nursing science" is used frequently today. But what do we mean by the phrase "nursing is a science" or the term "nursing science"? I hope we do not mean nursing practice is, or should become a science. Practice and science are two distinctly different processes with two different goals.

I had a stroke in 1972. If I have another catastrophic illness, or even if I just need health counseling, please don't get me a scientist, get me a good nurse. When I am ill or have a health problem of significance, I may need a physician, but I am also apt to need a person with particular interpersonal and procedural skills who has authentic knowledge from selected sciences. I need a person who can use that scientific knowledge and those skills in a compassionate and ethical manner in the interest of my health and comfort. Such a person with particular interpersonal and procedural skills, and with scientific knowledge and ethics, is what a nurse is.

Scientists are different. The scientist has a goal of discovering or producing knowledge in the form of theories or laws, or organizations of facts that have meaning, that make sense. Scientists seek to be objective, to control their biases, to minimize their individual or personal effect on an experiment.

Caring for patients may also require some objectivity, but it is also subjective. Caring involves one's person. Caring has a goal of beneficence, that is, doing good for other human beings. When I am a patient, I do not want to be viewed as an object of science. I want to be viewed as a unique, particular, perhaps even peculiar, individual who needs the ministrations and solace that caring, knowledgeable, compassionate nurses can provide. Practice requires the utilization of science, but it is not in itself science. Attention to the particulars of individuals, of states, and of settings are vital for effective practice. But effective practice also requires the use of some generalizations that are the products of science.

Excellent nursing practice is exquisite artistry. It is the artful selecting and fitting of the generalizations from science only as they are appropriate to a particular patient in a particular situation. Art is blending generalizations and particulars to create effective means to produce beneficence.

Theories are generalizations. Nursing theories are those generalizations that are necessary and useful in effective practice. Generalizations are the products of the two major processes of science: theory and research. Theory and research are the processes used to advance knowledge. Unfortunately, in nursing, we have been preoccupied with arguing about or learning methods. We have neglected, to an appalling degree, the substance of research while learning a process called research.

We have failed to ask what are significant knowledge questions that need to be researched. What do we need to have researched? How good is the knowledge we claim as the rationalization for our actions and decisions? Many of the untested theories or fragments of knowledge we have utilized as our knowledge base for practice have originated from views of humans, of families, or from general perspectives quite different form the values and orientations that have characterized nursing.

With concern for inadequacies in our knowledge, we have studied and emphasized how to do research. We have failed to specify what to research and why. We must correct this lack. We must specify what we need to know, what we need knowledge about. We must build a body of research that leads to an organized body of verified knowledge, the body of knowledge essential for responsible professional practice of nursing.

We lack a system of nursing knowledge. We have no clear cut idea of exactly what knowledge is needed as the base for effective practice. Variations in curricula attest to this. We are naive about the rigor or validity of the theories or rationales we use in practice though we think of ourselves as responsible professionals.

In the late 1800s a great discovery was made in medicine. Physicians came to realize their standard interventions were worthless and even harmful. In prescientific medicine bloodletting, purges, leeches, and the like were standard interventions. Perhaps our nursing interventions based on outmoded family theories or concepts such as sensory deprivation, outmoded theories about attitudes, segmented views of humans, and the like are equally worthless or perhaps even harmful. We may be using invalidated theories or be swayed by fads, charisma, or personal interests. How effective are our interventions? On what tested theories are they based?

What phenomena are the interventions intended to address, alter or change for the better, by nursing modalities? Where is any taxonomy of nursing interventions or nursing phenomena? We may agree that nursing phenomena are some class or classes of human responses or human behaviors in regard to health, but beyond this vague general idea, we have little specification. We tend to talk using general concepts, noble global phrases, and we have not yet begun to build a system of knowledge with nursing practice as the referent. We need to organize systems of concepts and relate these to researchable variables. We need to systematize or clarify our values and ethics, our concepts, our phenomena, and our practice goals and strategies.

We have long talked about meeting patients' needs. But what data do we collect to measure needs? How do we move from the abstract idea needs to observable realities we can systematically and reliably research?

Let me illustrate one way I've begun to move from ideas or concepts to observable data. Take the term nutrition. Patients, as all humans, need nutrition. Nutrition is a common human need mentioned in nursing schema. But how does one measure nutrition? What do nurses do to produce nutrition? One doesn't see nutrition. It is not something one can observe.

Nurses do observe patients' patterns of food ingestion. Patterns of food ingestion, what, how much, when, and how patients ingest, are things nurses can and do observe, and can and do have considerable impact on and responsibility for. For healthy, well, intact persons, nurses may have some responsibility and effect on food ingestion but so do many others. But for persons with special problems, such as liver disease, debility, strictures of the esophagus, bone marrow transplants, etc., nurses are often critically responsible for effective ingestion regardless of who prescribes or prepares what is to be ingested. Ingestion is observable. Nutrition, an idea, is not. How ingestion can be effected is often a nursing challenge and nursing responsibility. Patterns of ingestion are a phenomenon nurses can influence, and we can measure our influence. Other essentials for living can also be thought about as patterns of observable behavior rather than vague "needs." Observable behaviors can be researched.

I would like to share my first approximation for organizing nursing inquiry to eventually build a system of nursing knowledge and lead to

the specification of nursing phenomena and areas for nursing research. I will comment briefly on how different types of inquiry might
relate to practice. I think I will show why research or inquiry is essential for responsible practice of the professional quality our patients
and clients deserve.

My proposed organization includes several ways of knowing of
which science is only one. There are a variety of ways of knowing. You
can readily recognize differences between scientific knowledge, folk-
lore, personal, moral, or political knowledge, for example. For nursing
practice, there are four general types of knowledge that clearly are
essential. The four categories I find essential for practice are:

1. Scientific knowledge
2. History
3. Philosophy, and what I term
4. Nursing technologies

The fourth category, nursing technologies, includes interpersonal,
educative, procedural, and organizational techniques of various kinds.
Inquiry or research is needed in all areas, science, history, philosophy,
and the gamut of nursing technologies, and they all relate to practice.
Let me illustrate.

First, consider scientific knowledge. Much of what we use in practice is knowledge provided by fields such as anatomy, psychology, and
biology, which provide descriptions, and generalizations called theories or models that are used by nurses and others. Theories and
models from science give us understanding of the nature of things,
events, processes, and the like. The sciences from which we get some
knowledge for practice are not concerned with nor focused upon
nursing practice, however. Many decisions and actions in nursing practice require synthesis of theories or models across fields of science.
An illustration of this is in the prevention and treatment of decubitus
ulcers. We know to a considerable extent what causes decubiti or what
factors may be predisposing. We know decubiti are easier to prevent
than cure or heal. We are far from effective enough in either prevention or treatment of decubitus ulcers. We do not know why some
patients with predisposing conditions avoid getting decubiti while
others do not.

Another type of knowledge nurses need is nursing history. History
gives comprehensive understanding of events, eras, traditions or the

development of institutions, practices, or statuses. To understand why nursing practice has been disease centered in the main, but seems to be evolving to a health centering, one needs to know history. To understand why many nurses feel powerless, one needs to know history. To come to appreciate the great accomplishments and successes of nurses, one needs to know history. Why have we moved from functional assignments, to team nursing, to primary nursing? One needs to know history. With more knowledge of history we might reduce our tendency to repeat mistakes and generate problems for ourselves.

A third type of knowledge and inquiry is essential for nursing practice. It is philosophy. Philosophic inquiry seeks to clarify or organize existing knowledge, not develop new knowledge. Philosophy provides knowledge of ethics, of values, of foundations, and of roots. Philosophy provides knowledge of ethics, of values of foundations and of roots. Philosophy addresses comprehensive questions. There have been a few studies done by nurses as philosophers. One such study was a study of the meaning of suffering done by Kriedler (1979).

Kriedler explored meaning in suffering to articulate an approach in nursing intended to humanize the nurse's encounter with those who suffer. The approach offered an alternative to the need for self-control and control of others to protect against feelings of helplessness. The possibility of transcendence was discussed. This philosophical study has immediate usefulness for nursing practice. One might even wonder if transcendence as a human response could be considered as one phenomenon of interest to nurses. Philosophic studies have been done on empathy, health and healing, and ethics.

Norberg, a Swedish nurse, in conjunction with philosophers, identified ethical dilemmas that occur with nursing care of elderly patients with extreme dementia. Extreme dementia can produce a condition where spoon feeding is no longer possible or is very hazardous. One alternative is tube feeding, which may have to be forced. It can also be hazardous. Starvation is not acceptable. Nursing care of patients with extreme dementia is surely an overwhelming nursing challenge fraught with unavoidable dilemmas. Philosophical inquiry can clarify ethics and dilemmas.

A final general category of knowledge essential for effective nursing practice is that which I have labeled nursing technologies. Research in this category would have as its purpose the development, or testing, of the procedures, techniques, or the ways we do things in practice. Important sub-categories of techniques are interpersonal, mechanical, organizational, or educative.

An example of what I mean by mechanical or procedural techniques, or those having to do with nursing apparatuses or care procedures, is that provided from a follow-up on the situation of the Swedish nurse with patients with extreme dementia. A Swedish nurse visited our school last year, and I learned that Norberg, the nurse who had done the ethical dilemma study, had experimented with bottle feeding of her elderly patients and it seemed to be working. An innovative procedure may have resolved an ethical dilemma.

As responsible professionals, we must continually ask if our rationales are tested by research. Is our way of doing something the only or the best way? Are we simply rather unthinkingly following rote or tradition? Are our techniques really effective? Do they really produce quality results efficiently? Economically? Do our techniques make a significant difference? How do we know?

Responsible practice requires that we answer these questions with data. Unwarranted assumptions, good intentions, impressions, faith, and hope are not enough. Critical, systematic analysis, and evaluation of our knowledge and of our practice is an unavoidable professional responsibility.

Proof that our practices are effective is a kind of knowledge that gives one power and unlimited potential for effective persuasion. Knowledge and data are important sources of power. Let's get the facts through research. Let's examine our knowledge base for practice and improve it through inquiry where needed. Let's question, inquire, and develop our theory through research. Let's build a better future to add to a significant past through attention to the transmission, development, and utilization of knowledge.

REFERENCE

Kriedler, M.C. Meaning in suffering: A nursing dilemma (Doctoral dissertation, Columbia University Teachers College, 1978). *Dissertation Abstracts International*, 1979, *39*, 4813B (University Microfilms No. 79-09001)

8

Nursing Knowledge Development

EDITORS' INTRODUCTION

Doctoral forums in nursing had begun in the 1970s as an opportunity for faculty from the various doctoral programs to meet and deliberate issues. Ellis attended many of these annual forums and in 1984 was called upon to present this paper, which became a classic. In it, she delineates the types of nursing knowledge necessary for the discipline, making a distinction between the clinical science of nursing and other areas of nursing research. At this time in the development of the discipline, clinical nursing research was predominant.

Knowledge is something we all know about. In nursing, we have promoted nursing research and nursing theory development to advance and organize nursing knowledge. We have argued and advocated various methods, various concepts, and various theories and models, but we have had very little organization or cohesion in our efforts toward the development of nursing knowledge. We have a plethora of meanings for each of the highly abstract concepts deemed necessary for models or theories of nursing. We may agree that the essential terms are: nursing, client, health and environment. But what we agree

"Nursing Knowledge Development" presented June 21, 1984 at the National Forum on Doctoral Education, Denver, Colorado.

on are the words; we do not agree, except at the grandest abstract level, on the concept meanings of these words.

We have become preoccupied with highly abstract ideal types or ideologies while conducting research that produces fragments of data or findings which rarely are contributions to any cohesive system of knowledge that improves nurses' ability to care for clients. We are not effectively producing a system or body of knowledge that enhances practice or that expedites the education and socialization of generations of competent nurse practitioners and investigators. We have become conscious, conceptually, of the nature of nursing thinking, of the value of research and theory development, and we advocate methods for knowledge development. Nevertheless we have failed to attend to the structuring or organization of nursing knowledge though we have long spoken of a body of knowledge.

Knowledge acquisition and knowledge representation depends upon conceptual structuring and organization. Researchers in the field of artificial intelligence have clearly demonstrated that whatever knowledge is, it is not a string of data nor a bunch of facts. Congeries of tested hypotheses are also inadequate as knowledge. As one investigator in artificial intelligence has said, "no one can say what knowledge is exactly [and] 30 years of artificial intelligence research have not . . . improved upon 3,000 years of philosophy" (Waldrop, 1984, p. 1280). What artificial intelligence research *does* suggest, however, is that knowledge representation and acquisition are "so interwoven that they may as well be the same thing" (p. 1282) and that "whatever is going on inside our heads, is both highly structured and wonderfully reshapeable" (p. 1281). Similarly, a body of knowledge and a field of inquiry must be organized and structured, and both, by nature, are reshaped by research and theory development.

Knowledge structuring, except perhaps in the organization of curricula, is a neglected field in nursing. Donaldson and Crowley (1977) suggested approaches to structuring nursing knowledge and sketched out themes to identify our domain. We have done little to critique or advance the conception of nursing as a discipline. Perhaps it is because too few of us have attempted to study the nature of disciplines or to heighten our understanding of nursing as a discipline.

In our concern for nursing research and theory development we have made mistakes which have been generally detrimental for organizing knowledge or structuring knowledge development in the context of a discipline. In my view, these mistakes have been especially detrimental for doctoral education in nursing, for excellence in doctoral education requires conceptualization of nursing as a discipline. One mistake made was to argue processes to the neglect of systematic delineation of the *phenomena* of paramount importance to the discipline of nursing. By phenomena I mean *observable* facts or events of scientific interest that are susceptible of scientific description and explanation. I mean *observable* as distinguished from *concepts* which are mental images or *meanings*. We have confused ideations and observables. Even worse, we have dealt with concepts in isolation in some instances. We have failed to recognize that concepts are ideas or meanings. They are abstractions that have meaning *only* because they are a part of some cohesive system of concepts, or because they are specified by indicators or indexes that tie them to observables. A concept alone has no particular usefulness. A concept has meaning only because it is related to other concepts in some organization of concepts, in which case its meaning is a systemic or terminologic meaning that is lost if the concept is used out of context of its systemic meaning context. Concept meaning may arise from ties to empirical experience or observation with specification of the indicators or empirical referents for the concept. Nursing literature unfortunately is rampant with concepts not tied either to clearly delineated systems of concepts nor to empirical indicators. We use fragmented ideations with inadequate referents, and have neglected to specify the *phenomena* or observable things or events we need to explain. Theory development and research are processes to produce knowledge. We have argued about the processes, but have neglected specification, in terms of phenomena, of what it is that nurses need to know. We need to describe nursing in terms of the phenomena that nurses fix, alter or maintain through nursing modalities. For what nursing *phenomena* are our strategies of compensating, supporting, maintaining, counseling or educating the appropriate and necessary therapeutic actions? What alterable variables are our concern or what client or patient variables under what conditions may require nursing for stable maintenance? What is the subject matter of the discipline?

Another mistake we have made has been to espouse systems theories in general but to have failed to analyze nursing knowledge systematically in much detail or to systematically organize or advance that knowledge. It is my contention that one major source for our fragmentation, disagreements, polarities and endless frustrations, stems from the use of the one word *nursing* to name or label a profession, a process, an academic discipline, a social institution and a practice. When the word *nursing* is used, all too often the reader or listener must supply the meaning which may be that of profession, a distinctive clinical practice, a distinctive goal oriented process or even a scholarly discipline or field of inquiry. Though each of these meanings or *nursings* are related, the profession, the practice, the process and the discipline are four distinct entities and meanings. When we fail to make clear the meaning intended for a given use of the word *nursing* we produce confusion. This is especially a hazard when considering doctoral education where it is imperative to identify the nature of nursing as a discipline, as field of inquiry, and community of scholars concerned with knowledge development of a type called nursing.

Nursing knowledge, as distinct from nursing as a profession, nursing as a process or nursing education, must be organized and developed. It must be organized and developed to advance the nursing profession, to specify and clarify what practitioners need to process and why, and to expedite education in nursing.

Nursing as a profession or occupation is not my meaning of the word *nursing* here. That is because I am concerned with the organization of nursing knowledge. Nursing knowledge is of import in the three major activities for which nurses have responsibility, activities that we call nursing practice, nursing education, and nursing inquiry. The three are inextricably related, but for analysis and understanding, should be distinguished by their different processes. They are also different with respect to knowledge.

Nursing practice is predominately the *use* of knowledge. Nursing education involves the *transmission* of knowledge. Nursing inquiry is for the *development* and evaluation of nursing knowledge. Use, transmission or acquisition, and generation and testing of knowledge, are related or ought to be, but they are distinguishable and ought to be. Let me explain.

Nursing practice is the use of knowledge. It is the use of general knowledge, the use of nursing knowledge, of skills, and of self in the context of ethics and nursing values toward a goal of beneficence for clients. Though the various conceptualizations of nursing popular to-day are different in exactly how they specify the goals of nursing practice, the meanings of all such goals connote health for nursing clientele in some form, and all are *intended* beneficence. The benefi-cence intended is produced by nurses doing nursing with particular techniques and strategies focused upon health statuses, health poten-tials and health behaviors or responses, of individuals and groups. Beneficence for others, called patients or clients, is the raison d'etre, the goal, the justification, and the source of societal value, for nursing practice. Nursing practice is the only justification for the nursing pro-fession.

Knowledge for nursing practice entails many types of knowledge, moral, social, personal, and scientific at the very least. It also requires knowledge of particulars, of particular persons, or particular settings or situations, or of particular beliefs or cultures. But it is not the knowledge per se that produces beneficence. It is the artful, ethical *use* of knowledge that produces beneficence for others.

Nursing education exists to provide systems for the *transmission* and *acquisition* of knowledge in opportunities designed to produce the directed change or learning necessary to prepare nursing practi-tioners, administrators, and investigators. The knowledge to be trans-mitted or acquired is knowledge of self and others, knowledge of things and events in nature and in society, and the particular beliefs, values, skills and techniques necessary for professional functioning and being. In education, the processes of learning must be focal, and the immediate goal of nursing education is the preparation of nurses for practice, organization of practice, or for the advancement and organization of nursing knowledge. Nursing practice is the utilization of knowledge, some of which is distinctively nursing knowledge, for a goal of beneficence of nursing clientele. Nursing education is for the transmission or acquisition of knowledge toward the goal of prepared nurses. Of course, nursing practice must be the ultimate referent for nursing education, but we should not confuse educational processes and goals with those focal to and characteristic of beneficent clinical nursing practice.

Nursing inquiry is a third major activity for which nurses have responsibility. Nursing inquiry ought to have nursing practice as an ultimate referent, but nursing inquiry is very different from nursing practice. Nursing as a field of inquiry is a very different entity from nursing as a clinical practice. One obvious difference is the number of nurses who are engaged in and are concerned with clinical nursing practice compared to those who should or could focus upon nursing as a field of inquiry. This is not to say there are not scholars or investigators among the clinical experts in practice. It is to say that beneficence for clientele should be the primary goal of practice and nursing practice is the reason for the being of all else in nursing. The primary goals and processes for nursing inquiry are those necessary for the organization and development of knowledge, not those for the immediate beneficence of nursing clients. The processes for nursing inquiry will be *mastered* by the relatively few nurses who elect graduate education at the doctoral level. There are always exceptional individuals who make significant contributions and impact on their own, but as a probability, it is unlikely that nursing as field of inquiry will be advanced by those who have not studied nursing at an advanced level and engaged in a program of research to develop, test and organize nursing knowledge.

I do not intend in any lasting sense to separate nursing practice, nursing education or nursing inquiry. I merely wish to call attention to the fact that the word *nursing* has numerous meanings. It is both a noun and verb, discipline and practice, process and product. For the sake of nursing knowledge development and doctoral education development in nursing we ought to specify which meaning we intend when we use the word nursing. To that end, I suggest using the word nursing as an adjective so others can understand whether practice or field of inquiry or profession is intended. This is advocated when activities, processes, organizational entities and purposes differ as they do for nursing practice, nursing as academic or professional discipline and nursing as a profession.

Failure to recognize the distinctions has led to chaos in the multiple meanings one can find for the terms *nursing science, nursing theory,* or *discipline* in nursing literature. Ephemeral, diffuse meanings for these and other critical terms abound. Some articles on *nursing science* for example, are sheer gibberish because the term has no stable delineated meaning. Such ephemeral, diffuse meanings for key terms confound the challenging task that those of us in doctoral education in nursing must accept as responsibility, namely the organization and development of nursing knowledge, or the enhancement of knowledge application in the advancement of nursing practice.

If one accepts responsibility for nursing knowledge and its applicability, then I contend it is necessary to distinguish nursing as practice and nursing as a field of inquiry to produce and evaluate the knowledge basic to such practice.

The distinction helps one to understand what could be meant by the saying that nursing is both an art and a science. Nursing as a distinctive clinical practice is not a science, nor should it be. Nursing care patients or client's is not *doing* science or *"sciencing"* though it does require the use of scientific knowledge. Science as a process is intended to be objective, producing generalizations and facts. It does not need to be compassionate, humanistic, person centered, nor centered on a goal of health benefit. Nursing practice cannot be science. Science as product is fact, factual generalizations, models, or explanations. It is knowledge, not beneficence.

Nursing practice requires use of some generalizations from science, such as that of the need for oxygen for maintenance of human life. But nursing practice also requires certain technical skills including interpersonal ones and many others essential to effect comfort, life support, self maintenance, learning or recovery and all the other health benefits that nurses may produce. Scientific knowledge is not enough for skilled nursing practice. Knowledge of carbohydrate metabolism won't guarantee a nurse can assess the subtleties of a given patient slipping into diabetic acidosis. Nursing practice requires clinical acuity, sensitivity, and the artful fitting of particular means and ends for particular persons and situations. When I need a nurse, I want a caring, compassionate, skilled clinician. I do not want a scientist. I want a nurse with common sense, and with specialized knowledge and skilled techniques. I want a nurse who can use these for *my* benefit in a compassionate, clinically effective and ethical way for my health and welfare. Nursing as a clinical practice is not and should not be science, though it must, in part, entail the *use* of scientific explanations. Nursing practice at its best is probably more a matter of careful observation and listening, a matter of values, sensitivity, circumstances, and exquisite artistry than it is science. Explanatory theories from science may certainly be one source that contributes to the critical thinking of expert clinicians but that thinking is much more than is connoted by the phrase "apply theory." Critical thinking and expertise in nursing practice is bound in actions. Human thinking and action, as in nursing practice, are so interwoven and often are so spontaneous to situations, to particulars and to feedback from actions in situations, that *deliberate* selection and application of theory in some objectified, reasoned, analytical staging probably distorts what really happens in the mind of the expert practitioner.

In a book titled *The Reflective Practitioner* (Schon, 1983) illustrates by case analyses how professionals in five fields think in action. He also argues that academics in general have "a view of knowledge that fosters inattention to practical competence and professional artistry" (p. ii). Perhaps in our striving to become scientific, we in nursing have neglected the richness in the minds of expert clinicians as a source of nursing knowledge. "The human mind is fluid, mercurial, *non-linear,* continuously connecting and reconnecting, able to order itself and say, "Aha!" (Waldrop, 1984, p. 1282). In the incredible mind of the expert clinician, explanations or generalizations provided by scientists are but one source for acting and reacting, for appraising and reappraising, for caring, valuing, and being.

Distinguishing knowledge for nursing practice and nursing practice itself does enable one to contemplate the processes, the phenomena, and the perspective central to the organization of nursing inquiry toward a system or cohesive body of nursing knowledge. Organization of nursing as a discipline was started by Donaldson and Crowley (1977) with their paper on the structure of nursing as a discipline and with the comments and identification of issues added by McKay (1977). We have failed to move much beyond those papers. Perhaps too few of us have tried to understand the nature of disciplines or struggle with the nature of disciplines with clinical practice. Perhaps we have been consumed with issues of ideologies or methodology to the neglect of delineation of specific subject matter for the discipline.

The popular conceptual models of nursing do not help us much in the conceptualization of nursing as a discipline. Some models arose as attempts to conceptualize idealizations of and focus for nursing practice. When we rejected nursing as merely some list of tasks, activities, functions, roles, or problems, models supplied something to answer the plaguing question in theory development discussions or research symposia, "What is nursing?" Models useful for conceptualizing nursing as a practice have implications for nursing inquiry, and for the nature of knowledge a professional practitioner must have. They have not been particularly useful for nursing as a field of inquiry. They do not specify nursing phenomena nor significant research questions for the field. The models or theories are highly abstract, may serve to shape or develop practice, but are at best general orientations not the substance of nursing research.

Some conceptualizations of nursing arose to describe nursing as a practice for purposes of curriculum development in nursing. Some have begun to generate some research on some client behaviors but they have not produced a comprehensive knowledge system for nursing inquiry and are unrelated to much that is called nursing research.

A few conceptualizations of nursing have been presented as presuppositions or frameworks for development of scientific knowledge of life processes, or for providing the knowledge basic to a practice goal of assessing, maintaining or enhancing health statuses, health assets and health potentials of nursing clientele through the strategies long used and inherent in nursing practice. Even these are far short of serving as discipline matrix.

Specific nursing phenomena, the objects of empirical research have yet to be systematically delineated. At best they are delineated at the *concept* or *construct* level, but rarely at the empirical referent or phenomenal level. Terms such as *needs, nursing problems, health behaviors* are not labels for observable entities, nor is something such as *body image.* They are concepts that must be given meaning by linkage with other concepts especially that of *nursing,* and by linkage to empirical specifics. They must be linked in cohesive substantial theoretical systems if they are to be rendered useful for producing scientific knowledge for nursing. Even if we solve the pressing problems of linkages of abstractions and empirical realities, and of explicating contextual meanings from linkages of concepts in conceptual systems, and tie these to observables, we will not have produced all that is necessary for delineating nursing as a field of inquiry.

Nursing as a field of inquiry must be concerned with more than the facts or generalizations or explanations that nurses as scientists using the nursing perspective might produce. Science is but one of the types of knowledge that nurses need and that nurses must organize or generate.

There are at least four major types of knowledge for which nurses must assume responsibility for developing. All of the four types might be included in nursing as a field of inquiry, though not all nursing knowledge need be *produced* by nurses. Evaluation of the usefulness of knowledge for nursing purposes would seem to require evaluation by nurses, however.

To understand and advance the nursing profession, nursing practice, nursing education, and nursing as a field of inquiry, the following four types of knowledge need to be pursued: 1) scientific knowledge, 2) knowledge of the type called history, 3) knowledge of the type produced by philosophic inquiry, and, 4) nursing technology.

Let me elaborate. Scientific knowledge is that produced to answer what and why questions about things in the natural world. It is knowledge in the form of laws, such as the law of gravity or Boyles law, or axioms, or substantiated facts, generalizations and tested or testable theories or models such as the double helix of DNA. Few would deny that nursing practice requires scientific knowledge, though we cannot agree on exactly what specific scientific knowledge all nurses must have. Nor can we agree on what models of science, the theoretical, the classificatory or cataloguing, or the empirical inductive, we might follow. Perhaps we are evolving an innovative model implied by the term *clinical science* appearing in nursing literature. Until we know what we want to know about what phenomena, it is useless to debate methods. We ought to be specifying the substance or objects of inquiry which scientist nurses must study. We certainly need scientist nurses and scientific inquiry in nursing, but that is not all we need.

We need nurses who are historians. History produces comprehensive interpretations for understanding particular events, eras, traditions, institutions, statuses, or developments. Some history of nursing as social institution, profession, practice, or occupation can be produced by historians who are not nurses. However, there are many events, eras, institutions, statuses, ideas and developments that nurses need to know about to understand the nature of nursing, and why we are where we are, that may not be of interest to historians in general. There are also some matters of history for which nursing meanings may require the way of looking at things and deriving meanings that come from being a nurse. Certainly any history of ideas or of concept meanings in nursing requires familiarity with the jargon of nursing that nurses acquire.

Scientific inquiry has been an expectation of doctoral education in nursing that leads to the Ph.D. degree. It is implied by the term nursing science. Do we not need to be concerned also with history as a way of knowing and inquiring about nursing?

The third type of knowledge nurses must have is that produced from philosophical inquiry. Like history, philosophy produces knowledge that is comprehensive and integrative. The knowledge produced by philosophers is not that of fact, or of meanings from the discovery, organization or interpretations of *facts*. Knowledge produced by philosophers is the explication of *norms,* and of roots or foundations, of values and ethics. It may be the explication and justification of methods and goals. We need nurses who are philosophers to study ethics or moral norms and their roots and consequences. We need nurses who are philosophers to explicate and clarify the values inherent in the lasting existence and justification of nursing as a social institution. We need nurses who are philosophers to explicate and clarify the nature of theoretical thinking and conceptual structures in nursing practice and nursing inquiry. Scientist nurses need to know the roots of their approaches to inquiry and the history of science in nursing. Philosophic inquiry and knowledge from historians can contribute to the maturation of nursing as a field of inquiry and to the development of truly professional practitioners who value and build their heritage and noble traditions.

Doctoral education in nursing and the organization and development of nursing knowledge cannot be successful without cognizance of the purposes, methods and contributions to understanding nursing, of science, history and philosophy.

A fourth type of knowledge for which inquiry is needed is that which I classify as nursing technology. By nursing technology I mean the techniques required for effective clinical nursing practice. These include therapeutic interpersonal techniques essential to achieving nursing goals, the development or improvement of nursing procedures or apparatuses for nursing care, or of effective educative techniques or technologies for use with patients or clients. The list would also include organizational techniques, such as effective staffing patterns, or organizational innovations to effectively distribute, organize or create systems of nursing care services. Evaluation of the effectiveness of all of the various nursing techniques and nursing technology generally, is a responsibility of scholarly professional nurses. Nurse investigators must be involved in the development of nursing science and nursing technology. They must evaluate that nursing science and nursing technology in the context and actuality of nursing practice at some point. We also need to know a great deal more of the nature of artistry in nursing practice.

Some nurse investigators and scholars must do the work of history for nursing and still others must explicate and clarify moral norms, meanings, ways of knowing in nursing and nursing values.

We have spent many years advocating nursing research and theory development in nursing. We have produced little science or scientific theory and we have not produced an impressive cohesive body of nursing knowledge. It was sobering to re-read the words of Myrtle Irene Brown (1964) published twenty years ago in *Nursing Research*. She identified two questions that were imperative in 1964. The first question she posed then was "How far have we progressed through research toward the development of an integrated body of nursing theory?" (p. 109). Her second question was, "How can we determine if a research project has a theoretical framework that will make possible a contribution to scientific knowledge?" (p. 109).

The answer to the first question about progress through research toward an integrated body of nursing theory is probably "almost none," as it was twenty years ago. We *may* think we have a better grasp on the answer to the second question that speaks to the importance of a theoretical framework for significant scientific nursing research but this has not been demonstrated to my satisfaction when I read all of the abstracts of doctoral dissertations to be found under the heading *Health Sciences, Nursing* in *Dissertation Abstracts International* for 10 years ending July 1982. From reading these many abstracts one gets no hint of any organized concerted effort to develop a systematic body of knowledge for nursing practice. The collection of 10 years of abstracts of doctoral dissertations under the *Health Sciences, Nursing* did little to improve my understanding of nursing as a health science or as anything else. Appallingly few of the studies described by their abstracts were theoretically based or even cast in the context of a body or system of nursing knowledge. As faculty in doctoral programs in nursing what are we doing to contribute to a system of nursing knowledge?

Carper (1978) has identified four essential ways of knowing in nursing practice. How are these to be considered in relation to cohesive knowledge development in nursing? The further explication of nursing as a discipline is an imperative for doctoral education in this field.

REFERENCES

Brown, M.I. (1964). Research in the development of nursing theory. *Nursing Research, 13,* 109–112.

Carper, B. (1978). Fundamental patterns of knowing in nursing. *Advances in Nursing Science, 1*(1), 13–23.

Donaldson, S.K., & Crowley, D.M. (1977). Discipline of nursing: Structure and relationship to practice. *Communicating Nursing Research, 10,* 1–22.

McKay, R.P. (1977). Discussion: Discipline of nursing—Syntactical structure and relation with other disciplines and the profession of nursing. *Communicating Nursing Research, 10,* 23–30.

Schon, D.A. (1983). *The reflective practitioner.* New York: Basic Books.

Waldrop, M.M. (1984). The necessity of knowledge. *Science, 223,* 1279–1282.

9

Theory Development in Nursing: The State of the Art

EDITORS' INTRODUCTION

In this paper, Ellis described briefly the historical development of theory in nursing. The mid-1980s in nursing was a time when theory development was at its peak. Throughout this period of emphasis on nursing knowledge development, Ellis continued to raise questions about the meanings of our knowledge to nursing practice.

A BRIEF HISTORY OF THEORY DEVELOPMENT IN NURSING

For at least twenty years nurse scholars and scientists have been engaged in a theory development movement in nursing. My hypothesis is that the movement evolved for several reasons. A major root, or reason, was the evolution of research in nursing. A second possible stimulus was the abandonment, because of its inadequacy, of body

"Theory Development in Nursing: The State of the Art" was presented at the 50th Anniversary Celebration of the General Juif—Sir Mortimer Davis Hospital, Montreal, Canada.

systems or disease classifications as major curriculum organizers. During the 1950s in the U.S. curriculum structures in nursing began to become quite diverse as biological centricity yielded to increased attention to psychological, developmental, interpersonal, and social factors. Curriculum structures and content were changed as public health nursing became required, and as mental health concepts were systematically integrated. Language in nursing became increasingly conceptual as curricula were reorganized by developmental stages, as birth to death, or by nursing problems, arenas of action, or wellness to illness.

The shift to conceptual language was also due to the growth of research in nursing. The founding, in 1932, of the Association of Collegiate Schools of Nursing contained the root of this growth of nursing research. A goal of the Association of Collegiate Schools of Nursing was the promotion of nursing research. The Association was the root that produced the journal *Nursing Research,* which was established in 1952, though envisioned earlier. The need for nursing research was recognized rather early in the twentieth century but there were no scientist nurses to do the research until nurses began to study in doctoral programs to acquire the knowledge and skills to do research.

As nursing research started to grow in the second half of the twentieth century, there came compelling questions: The obvious question "What is nursing research?" led to the question "What is nursing?" It also led to questions about *what* should be researched, and *how* research should be done. Soon *how* to do research was the major focus.

Nurses who got their research training in the social or behavioral sciences, such as sociology or psychology, learned the theories in these fields. They came to know the linkage or reciprocal relationship between theory and research. In the U.S., as nurse scientists grew in number, conferences on nursing research or nursing theory development began. These began the nucleus for communities of nurse scientists. Previously nursing groups of scholars were educationists.

Major basic curriculum shifts, the shift in focus of graduate programs in nursing from functional preparation to clinical preparation and introduction to research, coupled with the growth in numbers of nurses with research training and a general shift in nursing language from the concrete and procedural to the conceptual, inevitably and naturally produced the theory development movement in nursing.

STATE OF THE ART IN
THEORY DEVELOPMENT IN NURSING

My assignment for today was to comment on theory development in nursing in terms of the state of the art. I will do so by commenting on where we are, and on where we are not, knowing that we seem to have recognized some imperatives as to how to go forward. First, let me describe where we are.

Theory Development in Nursing: Where We Are

The title given me for this occasion should be noted. It characterizes theory development as an art. It is art; it is also a part of science as process. The words *art* and *science* each have multiple meanings. The word *art* means: knack, *skill in performance acquired by experience or study,* human ingenuity or contrivance, a branch of learning, and a number of other things. The meanings I delineated all seem to be meanings relevant to theory development in nursing.

Art is closely linked to science in art's meaning of general principles of a branch of learning. *Science* as a term means both science as process and science as product. Science as process means a way of seeking a particular kind of knowledge. The seeking is done by means of research processes. These are the processes for discovery, and for testing the theoretical formulations arising from discoveries. They are the processes for formulating testable theories, laws, axioms or generalizations. Theory development is the name for the processes which go with, and are reciprocal with, research processes. Science as product is factual knowledge or testable theoretical formulations that can be communicated, used and evaluated by others. Science is knowledge produced by processes that are made public, can be clearly explicated, and can be judged against agreed upon criteria. Scientific knowledge is that set forth in the form of laws, as the laws of gravity, or

Boyle's law; axioms; or organizations, or sets, of statements that are useful for prediction or explanation. Scientific theories and generalizations are the products produced by research and theory development processes.

My first observation on the state of the art of theory development in nursing is that we have produced little that warrants consideration as scientific theory. We *have* become aware of science as a process. We have recognized that facts by themselves have no meaning. Facts must be organized and interpreted by theorizing, by interpretations and by linkages with other facts so they *make sense.* Theories make sense from facts and data.

It has taken some time for us to begin to learn the terminologic language of science. In fact, we are still struggling with this. Failure to understand scientific processes as a great deal more than simplistically delineated procedural problem solving, has been a major source of our failure to reap great benefit for nursing from the research activities of nurses.

We early recognized the need for research so we began to learn and teach one method of *how* to do it. We attempt to teach how to do it, but we have not clearly identified what *it* is. The *what* and *why* in nursing for which theory and research is needed is not explicated clearly.

It is a puzzle to me why it is we nurses, as practitioners or as educators, scholars or researchers, seem to expend our efforts on exalting *processes.* Perhaps it is because historically *nursing* has been seen as a practical doing, a doing learned by doing. We have lately shifted from sole emphasis on procedures, a view which seemed to characterize early 20th Century nursing. But perhaps the shift is more illusory than substantive. Our emphasis on processes is still an emphasis on the steps or ways to do something. That could be useful were it not at the expense of neglect of the formulation and clear delineations of what to process, what to question or what to illuminate for what purposes. Much has been written on nursing process. We have almost nothing on the *phenomena* that are focal for nursing. We have not specified the things for which the process is useful, or *what the process is to accomplish* except in some grand abstract terms such as client health or welfare. Similarly we have had texts on nursing research for 25 years, mostly texts on how to do it, but as yet almost nothing on *what* to research, or what the significant questions or phenomena are for which the research process is needed.

Unfortunately, the same can be said for theory development except that we do not have a great deal yet that thoroughly illuminates all aspects of the processes for theory development and we again have not gotten organized clearly what it is we need to know, about what phenomena, that *would* be supplied if we knew how to develop theory and go about it.

Some of the possible reasons one can offer to explain the state I've just described might be we feel we must be doers, do not consider ourselves as nurses to be theoretical thinkers, and perhaps consider that being concerned with science, or being scientists, threatens the humanitarianism with which nursing has been identified. Other reasons might be our attention and preoccupation with learning or debating *methods* and *definitions of terms* such as *theory, model, concept, paradigm or metaparadigm* before conceptualizing nursing as a practice or nursing as a field of inquiry.

As we began to emphasize nursing research, we had to rely on experts such as statisticians or scientists in other fields to teach us how to do research and to develop theory. We have relied on experts from other fields to a considerable extent perhaps at the expense of doing some hard thinking ourselves. Early in the theory development movement the term *practice theory* was introduced. In 1964, Wald and Leonard, (1964, p. 311) in an article entitled "Toward Development of Nursing Practice Theory," described practice theory as that theory which would supply the "cause and effect understanding" necessary for effective nursing actions in practice. They considered that nurses' actions which have the intent to achieve "changes in patient's responses to illness, to hospitalization, to the medical regimen, and changes in the patient's ability to utilize health measures" (p. 311) had to be based upon knowing, in a cause and effect understanding, what was likely to be effective in causing *desired* change. It is clear that Wald and Leonard were arguing for theories of the form called causal process theory. It is also clear that by the term *nursing practice theory* they were not meaning some exotic, or unique to nursing, *type or form* of theory. They were arguing for causal rather than descriptive theory. Causal process theory is one form of scientific theory. What they deemed distinctive about *nursing* causal theories was the subject matter not the form. Nursing theories, in their meaning, were causal theories to provide the understanding for formulating effective actions. Actions meant were those to produce desired changes in patients responses through nursing practices. Descriptive theory would not suffice. Theories also were to be theories restricted to the use of causal variables that could be manipulated by the practitioner in nursing. In 1984, twenty years later, a symposium on explanatory knowledge in nursing was part of the program of the Seventeenth Annual Conference of WICHEN and the Western Society for Research in Nursing. The 1984 symposium indicated to me how we have failed to utilize the wisdom of Wald and Leonard. We are still debating or arguing *form* or *type* of theory and have not improved much on what to theorize about; we are now saying "human responses" instead of patients' responses but that is not a great deal of progress for 20 years.

A paper by Dickoff and James (1968) at a 1967 symposium on theory development, and their 1968 paper with Wiedenbach (Dickoff, James & Wiedenbach, 1968) on "Theory in a Practice Discipline," began to diffuse the meaning of the term *practice theory.* The papers also deflected attention from causal process theory or *forms* of theory to *levels* of theory, and introduced the idea of *prescriptive* theory. These papers were a catalyst in evoking conceptualizations of nursing in terms of goal or goals and in terms of processes rather than a list of tasks or activities, or functions, or roles. It still remains debatable as to what is meant by the terms *practice theory* or *prescriptive theory.* Beckstrand, in 1980, considered Dickoff, James and Wiedenbach (1968) to have meant practice theory to be something other than scientific theory. Practice theory has also come to mean a conception of nursing practice or characterization of nursing practice (Collins, R. J., & Fielder, J. H., 1981).

As we have become confused about what we mean by theory, and have argued forms or levels of theory, we have begun to use the terms *model, paradigm, metaparadigm, conceptual framework, theoretical framework,* and *conceptual model.* I do not intend to sort these out or try to define the terms. My refusal to even try to do this is because the ambiguities and proliferation or shifts in terminology are more a comment on the state of the art of theory development in nursing than a matter of definition. Our confusion is more than a

matter of definition or meaning of terms. The ambiguities and confusion arising from multiple meanings of abstract terms, compounded
by relative naivete about the nature of science, and what we intend to
mean by the term *nursing science,* does lead me to one observation
that may provide a beginning for untangling some of the confusion.

It is my contention that it is useless to try to fix a single meaning for
terms such as *model* or *theory.* The terms are used interchangeably.
They must be understood in context. They mean what a given author
means them to mean. It *is* essential to understand what the cognitive
or conceptual schema actually is that is labelled *theory* or *model.*
What it is, and what it is useful for, is what is critical, not what it is
called. What something actually is and for what it can be used has not
been attended to sufficiently in theory development in nursing.

A serious consequence of this has been failure to distinguish between models of actual "ises" and models of "oughts." Let me illustrate. Scientific models, such as those of the DNA double helix or
Krebs' cycle, are scientists' models of how they conceive actual natural
entities or biological processes to be. They schematically represent
conceptions of actualities. They are explanatory representations to
account for phenomena. They are heuristic for further scientific research and theorizing in the search for prediction, control or explanation of natural phenomena. (Natural phenomena may be things,
events and processes.) Lets call this type of theory or model "Explainers." They are instruments for causal process theory or for the seeking
of scientific laws, or factual generalizations. They are abstracted representations of nature as it is thought to be, or are representations of
how we think things *do* occur.

Conceptual models in nursing are not models that represent nursing as it now actually is or has been. They are models of envisioned
ideals. They are statements of how nursing *should* or *ought* to be
conceived or thought about. Practice theory, when it means a conceptualization or characterization of nursing as it might be conceived, or
ought to be conceived, and grand theories or conceptual models of
nursing are "Shapers." They are ideologies, or *visionary* theorizing
and not testable scientific theories.

Our failure to distinguish "explainers" of existing actualities, and
visionary ideological "shapers" for revising how we *should* think
about nursing, has been a major factor in our lack of great progress in

theory development in nursing. Some efforts have been directed to attempts to "test" by research, or to validate through research processes, "Shapes" which are ideologies or ideals not naturally occurring existing things, events or processes. Conceptual models or "Shapes" in nursing have almost become principalities to be defended or ideas to be popularized, or voted upon. Scientific models or theories are put forth as tentative "best" approximations or explanations or how actual natural entities are or why they occur. Such explainer theories are set forth to be tested, or revised by continuing research to augment the data that triggered their formulation.

Ideologies are belief systems expressing values and orientations. As shapers of thinking, as situation producers, as facilitators of conceptual thinking in nursing, and as orientations for nurses to think about what they could be about, and why, such shapers may serve as orientations to shape nursing practice and organize it. As ideals, they may shape changes in nursing curricula. The shapers may be orienting frameworks for nursing research. Shapers are useful as general orientations. It is, however, essential that we recognize the differences between scientific "explainers" and nursing "shapers." We have not always done so. We have evidence that nurses tend to confuse models of natural actualities, as developed by scientists and models of nursing as we think it *should* be conceived and as we would like to make it become. Shapers are not models to be tested by scientific processes. They are not products from science. They are important conceptualizations for shaping the future. They should not be "sold" by propaganda or popularity polls, or voted upon. Nor should they be mandated by authorities. They should be examined for their premises, their implicit values, their social congruence and contribution. They should be studied for their adequacy, their logic, and their usefulness.

In our present state of confusion about what nursing theories or models are, we have the absurdity of a number of highly abstract "Shaper" type models which have not produced much except general orientations. Simultaneously, we have atheoretical research by nurses. Or we have nurse researchers engage in disparate bits of research not related, and not reflecting any clearly articulated nursing framework.

As a consequence, we cannot point to any *cohesive* growing body of nursing knowledge. We have not produced much scientific theory.

Though we cannot be satisfied by the rate of progress, and though we lack the clear identity of a community of scholars, we are *not* where we were before the theory development movement began. Much good has come from our various efforts in theory development.

First, we have a heightened awareness of how we think as *nurses,* and we are sharing how we think about nursing theoretically. This has value because "a profession's service to society is an intellectual one" (Johnson, 1974, p.372). As responsible nurses we must examine and reexamine how we acquire and represent knowledge and constantly question the state and adequacy of our knowledge. The societal value of our contribution to peoples health depends upon that adequacy. Our attention to the continuities and commonalities in the various conceptual models of nursing, as well as the differences, has been rewarding. There is great agreement as to the modalities or strategies that characterize nursing as a practice. Nursing is generally seen as person oriented. There is agreement that client being and well being are to be maintained or enhanced by the strategies of compensations, support, counsel, learning, appraisal, and monitoring. There is great agreement that meaning in nursing comes from the meaning and linkages of the terms *person or client, nursing, health,* and *environment.* We agree on language, though exactly what the meaning of each of those terms is to be and how *client* and *environment* are linked vis-à-vis the focus, and strategy of action, of the nurse, varies from model to model. We do agree nursing has to do with clients responses and behaviors, thoughts and feelings, and physical states, relevant to health. It is clear we agree that maintenance of person is vital as well as body. We agree that nursing has to do with how people behave in the interests of their own health. All these agreements serve as a very useful dynamic answer to the question repeatedly posed very early in the theory development movement: "What is nursing?" The answer is dynamic because it is constantly up-dated, examined, clarified, and questioned. We are now conceptualizing nursing as goal-oriented. We are consciously attending to what we need to accomplish and not merely concerned with procedures or processes, (the how to do somethings) as ends in themselves. We are also much more aware of what we need to do to accomplish our goals. We are asking better questions. We can't be satisfied nor complaisant, but there is much to appreciate.

From the theory development activities we have recognized the importance of *concepts* as units of thought, and have begun to address the need for cohesive *systems* of concepts (Kim, 1983). Increasingly a few nurses are engaging in concept analysis and concept clarification. Such activity, vitally needed, will move us from being performing parrots talking noble global slogans to the effective relating of our concepts to meaningful practice experiential data.

As a result of our heightened awareness of the importance of concepts, and of meanings dependent upon relationships among concepts, several methodological issues have been identified. One is evident in the current debates about the relative value of quantitative methods. What is at issue is whether the significant questions for nursing research, and the appropriate, for nursing, perspective on the nature of our clientele, fit the striving for objectivity characteristic of a dominant view of science. At issue is whether given the nature of nursing and nursing clientele, human to human subjectivity offers better potential for generating important nursing knowledge. The debate is healthy, but a dialectic, or exchange of reasoning that is not aimed at polarizing and vehemently defending a single view should be sought. It is useless to defend poles when it is clear that both objective and subjective methods are relevant for nursing phenomena. We need to define or delineate the appropriate phenomena, the significant questions, the *nursing* questions and framework, *then* select or devise methods appropriate for the question.

In nursing, we have a tendency to defend rather than explicate, or reason. We need to identify not only issues, but what is *at* issue in the issue. Sometimes when what is *at* issue is clearly identified, it is possible to create the synthesis that improves the whole or creates a useful new way of seeing things. If synthesis is not possible, at least knowing what is *at* issue sharpens the area for further study, identifies the further evidence needed, or makes clear that resolution or agreement is not possible because it is an opinion matter that depends on grand perspective. Some of our debates or pole defending is much like the uselessness of debating whether a glass is half-full or half empty. Why one notices the glass, why one is considering the question, and one's general point of view, will affect one's answer. Research won't solve the problem. Opposite views and other polarities than those on method are evident in theory development in nursing. There are con-

ceptual models that view the environment as fraught with stress. Nursing then is viewed as helping clients successfully defend against stress.
Other models consider the environment to be in a symbiotic relationship to humans. These are opinions. Neither debate nor research will
give us final truth. It is a matter of opinion and focus not a matter of
science.

It has been provocative to have such alternate views offered in the
various models in nursing. It can stimulate healthy growth and clarification in our orienting thinking. It can do this *if* we avoid the tendency to defend, to line up band wagons, and become followers or
promoters rather than a community of scholars. Theory development
depends upon the healthy challenge, useful critiques, and stimulation,
of scholarly colleagues. We have some of that in nursing, but it must
flourish for real advancement of knowledge. We have the choice. We
can choose endless debate or healthy dialectic. We can respond to
charisma, personal loyalty, preferences of authorities, etc. or we can
act as scholars dealing with intellectual matters by reasoning, consideration of evidence, values, and consequences. Theory development
in nursing in the last twenty years may not have produced much
scientific theory, but it is beginning to create a community of scholars.
It has also been beneficial as it has served to identify some imperatives for the future.

THEORY DEVELOPMENT IN NURSING: IMPERATIVES FOR THE FUTURE

The development of nursing research, the acceleration of doctoral
education for nurses, and of research training, plunged us into theory
development in nursing.

From all this came the imperative to attend to the nature of nursing
as a discipline. Donaldson and Crowley's (1978) paper on nursing as a
discipline was a start in identifying the general domain of nursing
inquiry. They identified the domain from the persistent themes they
found evidenced in writings of nurses who had attempted to express
the essence of nursing. Donaldson & Crowley also discussed the usefulness of viewing nursing practice, and nursing as a discipline, as

highly related, but separate, entities. They identified the necessity of philosophic inquiry and of the historical method in consideration of nursing as a discipline. We seem so preoccupied with the trappings, rituals, and pet methods of science, we have done little to carry further what Donaldson & Crowley started. Consideration of nursing as a discipline needs to be pursued. That is one path we have come upon that needs to be followed further and explored.

Disciplines are characterized by a domain of phenomena. Domain and phenomena identify the subject matter for inquiry by the scholars or investigators in that field. Disciplines also have structure or conceptual principles of inquiry. Structure is in part "the body of imposed conceptions which define the investigated subject matter of that discipline and control its inquiries "(Schwab, 1962, p. 199). The current conceptual models serve some purpose in the general identification of the domain of nursing as a discipline. But we have barely begun to specify the phenomena within the domain. Identification of nursing phenomena has not been done. We have not clearly specified the observable actualities or client manifestations, for which, actions of nurses, as practitioners, are necessary, beneficial and of central focus. Identification of phenomena is a second imperative. At both the *concept* and the *phenomena* level, we need taxonomies, topologies or some other form, for organizing the "things" nurses "fix," or the "things" nurses maintain or enhance. Problem lists, lists of nursing diagnoses, and concepts one by one, have been offered, but without attention or explication of the premises, presuppositions, the theoretical framework, the conception of nursing practice, or the frame of knowledge to which they relate or from which they were derived. The social congruence, social utility and social significance of lists of problems or concepts has not always been made explicit. Nursing practice is a contribution to society and therefore must be accountable to that society (Johnson, 1974). Theories for nursing practice or conceptual models of nursing are not useful if they ignore social congruence and social significance as contextual imperatives.

If one accepts that nursing research and nursing theory development must ultimately have some relationship to nursing as a practice, then on conceptualization of that practice, as the researcher or developer of theory conceives it, is an implicit premise. It would be useful if theorists made their premises explicit.

A final imperative for theory development in nursing that has emerged is the necessity of testing the applicability and usefulness of theories in the actualities of practice. Coupled with this imperative is the need to create better mechanisms for communication and colleagueship, for the good of nursing, among scientist or scholar nurses and practitioners. It would be ideal if every nurse could be simultaneously expert practitioner, brilliant scientist, great humanitarian, noble statesperson, and dedicated scholar. Lacking realization of this impossible dream, we need each other.

Theory development in nursing is alive and growing. It needs some nurturing; perhaps, and some fertilization. It may be helped by strategic pruning and selective branching for stronger growth.

We have always known nursing requires a lot of thinking. Now we are growing aware of *how* we think and what we think or need to think about to meet our professional responsibility through nursing knowledge development by research and theory development.

REFERENCES

Beckstrand, J. (1980). A critique of several conceptions of practice theory in nursing. *Research in Nursing and Health, 3,* 69–79

Collins, R. J., & Fielder, J. H. (1981). Beckstrand's concept of practice theory: A critique. *Research in Nursing and Health, 4,* 317–321.

Dickoff, J., & James, P. (1968). A theory of theories: A position paper. *Nursing Research, 17,* 197–203.

Dickoff, J., James, P., & Wiedenbach, E. (1968). Theory in a practice discipline. *Nursing Research, 17,* 415–435, 545–554.

Donaldson, S. K., & Crowley, D. M. (1978). The discipline of nursing. *Nursing Outlook, 26,* 113–120.

Johnson, D. E. (1974). Development of theory: A requisite for nursing as a primary health profession. *Nursing Research, 23,* 372–377.

Kim, H. S. (1983). *The nature of theoretical thinking in nursing.* Norwalk, CT: Appleton-Century-Crofts.

Schwab, J. J. (1962). The concept of the structure of a discipline. *Educational Record, 43,* 197–205.

Wald, F. S., & Leonard, R. C. (1964). Towards development of nursing theory. *Nursing Research, 13,* 309–313

10

Nursing Scholarship and Nursing Practice

EDITORS' INTRODUCTION

Ellis continued to emphasize the link between nursing science and professional practice. It should be noted that this was a time when the disciplinary leaders were struggling with the integration of science and practice. Many doctoral programs in nursing had begun to emphasize research without a direct link to practice. Although clinical research was dominant, questions were raised about the relationships between basic and applied (clinical) research.

Honor the physicians for the need thou hast of them. . . . You are ignorant of maladies which seem to you to be the same. You must endeavor particularly to remember and observe their method of treating the sick, so that when you will be in the villages or any other place in which there is no doctor, you may render yourself useful by applying their method. You ought therefore to instruct yourselves, so as to know in what case it is necessary to bleed in the arm or in the foot. What quantity of blood you should take on each occasion; when to apply the cupping glasses. Learn also the different remedies necessary to be used in the various kinds of diseases and the proper time and manner of administering them. All this is very necessary for you and you will do a

Unpublished paper "Nursing Scholarship and Nursing Practice" written October 8, 1984.

great deal of good when you are well instructed in it. I think it is very essential that you should have some conferences with one another on this subject in the form of catechism. (Austin, 1957, pp. 142–143).

Thus wrote St. Vincent de Paul to the Daughters of Charity at the Hotel Dieu of Paris in the 17th Century. Rote learning, mimicry of physicians, and catechism were the sources of knowledge for nursing practice before the advent of formal education for nurses. Folk lore undoubtedly also was relied upon. Even with the development of the Nightingale School at St. Thomas' Hospital in London in 1860, obedience to authorities, reliance on physicians as knowledge authorities, and a view of nursing as prescribed tasks or procedures was perpetuated. Nightingale believed nurses' training was best done in a hospital in which there was medical research, but scholarship and research were not expected of nurses. The Nightingale School curriculum did include lectures by physicians on the sciences, such as the chemistry of air and food and anatomy and physiology. Nurses were expected to be users of science, and to understand the rationales for why they should do procedures and observations in specified ways.

Sciences and the works of selected scientists were evident as recommended content for teachers and students of nursing in the first *Standard Curriculum for Schools of Nursing* published in 1917 by the National League for Nursing Education. The curriculum recommended emphasized theoretical foundations as essential for really good practical work, and the need for more than scattered fragments of scientific knowledge. Scientific inquiry was valued as was the experimental work atmosphere of large teaching hospitals. Laboratory work in dietetics and sciences was detailed. One objective of the anatomy and physiology course was to discourage haphazard and pseudoscientific thinking about the body and its functions. Practice in the correct use of scientific terms, and training in observation to arouse interest in scientific work was recommended. A rationalized approach to nursing activities and procedures was advocated, and students were to seek out reasons, and to systematize and classify ideas.

Concern for research in nursing was very evident in the establishment of the Association of Collegiate Schools of Nursing in 1933. This organization, a constituent member of the American Council on Edu-

cation, had as one of its purposes or goals, the encouraging of research. It is from this Association of Collegiate Schools of Nursing that
the seed for the journal Nursing Research came. The journal appeared
in 1952 to inform nurses of the results of scientific studies in nursing
and to promote research in nursing.

Although one can find occasional research studies pertaining to
patient care or nursing technologies in the early 20th Century
(Gortner & Nahm, 1977), it was not until the 1950s that nursing
research began to be emphasized. Supply and demand studies of
nurses and nursing education were notable, but the nurse as scientist
or researcher was not the expected.

In her foreword to Bridgeman's *Collegiate Education for Nursing*,
E. L. Brown (1953) did emphasize the importance of professional
education for nurses who must assume responsibility for the quality
of the social functions that nurses perform. One of these functions for
which nurses were responsible, according to Brown, was research.

A major catalyst in the development of nursing research was the
series of studies of nursing functions by the American Nurses' Association in the fifties. These studies created a nationwide focus on research among nurses. The studies were organized by a master plan,
and state nursing associations, universities, and a variety of social
scientists as investigators, became involved in studies of nurses and
nursing as practiced. This alliance between nurses and social scientists, and a concomitant emphasis on mental health, which resulted in
investigation by psychiatric nurses, resulted in nurses becoming part-
ners in research with social scientists (Gortner, 1980). It also perpetuated the tendency to treat nurses as the objects of research rather
than patients or patient phenomena.

In 1955, from voluntary assessments of the general membership,
the American Nurses' Association created the American Nurses'
Foundation, Inc. The foundation was established to support and fund
nursing research. Nursing was unique among professions in taxing its
general membership to support research.

Another source for funding nursing research was the development
of extramural research support by the Division of Nursing Resources
in the United States Public Health Service, and the creation of a
Research Grant and Fellowship Branch in 1954. Fellowships became
available to enable nurses to study for research training. In 1959,

Vreeland, first chief of the Research Grants and Fellowship Branch, listed studies that should be done (Gortner & Nahm, 1977), which included studies of nursing practice and patient care.

Preparation for nursing research among nurses was augmented by the explosion of master's programs in nursing in the fifties and the shift at the end of the fifties to clinical majors and an introduction to research processes.

From the American Nurses' Association program of studies of nursing functions, which involved numbers of nurses in financial support of research, and underscored the need for some nurses to be educationally prepared to do research, came a general acceptance of nursing research as a professional responsibility.

In 1958 the first book on nursing research was published, A. F. Brown's *Research in Nursing*. The book discussed research and the research processes. Included in an appendix was a list of 108 nurses known to have an earned doctorate. Approximately 90% of those listed had studied in the field of education; few were fundamentally scientists.

It can be said that by 1960 resources for nursing research were being marshalled. Some nurses were acquiring competency as investigators, research funding was becoming available, and nurse educators, professional organizations, and the federal Division of Nursing were promoting nursing research and organizing conferences to present or discuss nursing research. A goal of research to produce the body of knowledge necessary for professional practice in nursing was accepted. That such a goal has not been realized can be explained by a number of factors.

Once research was accepted as a necessary professional responsibility, unfortunately attention was directed primarily to discussion and learning research processes or the how to do it of research. Organized delineation of the substantive structure of nursing as a field of inquiry was neglected. General identification of types of studies of inquiry was neglected. General identification of types of studies needed were sometimes offered, but the subject matter of nursing as a field of inquiry was not specified except in generalities.

In part, the neglect arose from the fact that the one term *nursing* was used for nursing practice, nursing education, and the nursing profession. Nursing research simply meant research in any of these areas. A few nurse scientists did clinical research (Abdellah, 1970) but measurement and conceptual problems made the work hard. Efforts of individual researchers were noteworthy, but there was little concerted effort to identify nursing as a distinctive field of inquiry and great disagreement as to how to proceed with nursing research given the immensity and complexity of nursing.

Wald and Leonard (1964) noted early the inadequacies in development of a scientific body of knowledge for nursing practice. They attributed the failure to the use by nurses of the aims and methods of educational research, or to attempts to apply aims or methods of basic sciences to problems of nursing care of patients. Nurses tended to use the orientations of other fields, which rarely produced knowledge deemed vital to the nurse in practice. Wald and Leonard argued for empirical studies in nursing practice to develop hypotheses from observations in actual clinical nursing practice. Nurses who were not satisfied with nursing practice as it was, rejected study of actual practice as a desirable approach and argued for grand conceptualizations and theoretical approaches.

Wald and Leonard did not intend that practice as it actually was should be accepted without question. Their thesis was that patient phenomena in clinical nursing that nurses, as practitioners, might affect for good should be the subject matter for nursing research and theory development in nursing. Orem's (1979) applied nursing sciences' object: the realities that nurses observe and regulate as nurses, is similar in meaning.

By *theory*, Wald and Leonard meant scientific causal theories restricted to the use of causal variables that could be manipulated by nurses using modalities. They identified as problems in the development of nursing practice theory and research, traditional nurse passivity, and dependence on physicians or authorities in other disciplines, rather than nurses exercising intellect and creativity. Another element was the lack of appropriate research methods for clinical research in nursing, and a general naiveté about research.

At nursing research and theory development conferences in the sixties three compelling questions persisted. The questions were, "What is nursing?," "What is nursing research?," and "What is nursing theory?" The questions persisted because they were not answered satisfactorily. Nurse scientists who learned research in fundamental sciences or fields used by nurses preferred to continue research in the idiom of their doctoral fields, failed to continue as researchers as they took positions as nursing education administrators, or experienced some delays and difficulties in evolving collaboration with expert practitioners or becoming immersed in the actualities of patient phenomena. Every nurse ideally should be expert practitioner, brilliant scientist, great humanitarian, noble statesperson, and dedicated scholar. Lacking this ideal, collaboration of practitioner and researcher is needed. The demands of practice and of research and scholarship are each great. Too often the two worlds of nursing are far apart.

Nursing curricula reflect some lack of agreement as to the nature of nursing. Where once biological centricity characterized nursing curricula, paralleling developments in medical sciences, about 1950, increased attention was given to psychological, developmental, interpersonal, and social factors. Language in nursing became more conceptual than observational. As concepts became focal, lists of discrete concepts multiplied. Unfortunately, concepts in isolation do not comprise a body of knowledge. Too often the meanings of concepts were not derived from linkages to nursing strategies, goals, or to patient observables or phenomena. Nurses adopted concepts or theories, or parts of theories, poorly related to empirical indicators in the world of nursing practice. Nurse scientists who learned research in social or behavioral sciences often used theories and concepts of these fields, or taught these rather than nursing.

Conferences on research or theory development processes became forums for arguments about methods or about definitions of *theory* or of *nursing research*. The *what* and *why* in nursing for which the processes of research and theory construction were needed were not explicated.

Nurses exalted processes. Texts on nursing research were mostly texts on how to do it. There is yet almost nothing on what phenomena need to be researched, or on the significant questions for which the research process is needed.

Early in the research and theory development movements some nurses thought that concern with science threatened the humanitarianism with which nursing has been identified. As developing scientists, nurses relied heavily on experts from other fields. Instead of heeding the wisdom of Wald and Leonard (1964), in 1984 nurses are still debating forms, types, levels, and definitions of *theory* (see for example Beckstrand, 1980; Collins & Fielder, 1981; Beckstrand, 1984) and research methods (Munhall, 1982; Silva and Rothbart, 1984). Helpful as the debates are in the clarification of issues in knowledge development in nursing, they have led to discussions *about* science, and do not seem to have accelerated the actual development of much nursing science.

The term *practice theory* for Wald and Leonard (1964) meant causal theory about nursing phenomena. Diffusion of the meaning of the term came with Dickhoff, James, and Wiedenbach (1968). Practice theory for these authors meant four levels of theory including prescriptive theory and a conception of nursing practice. Subsequent confusion as to the meaning of *practice theory,* and *prescriptive theory* has vitiated progress in production of research based on tested theory that is meaningful for improvement of nursing practice.

It has been helpful to conceive of nursing practice in terms of goals and strategies rather than as a list of activities, procedures, functions, or roles. Dickhoff, James, and Wiedenbach emphasized goal conceptualization and probably accelerated nurses attention to explicating conceptual models of nursing. The diffuse meanings for the term *theory,* however, led to confusion between nursing models that are ideologies or visionary theorizing as to how nursing should be conceived, or are abstract representations of humans as nurses ought to view them, and explanatory theories developed to explain observable human responses that nurses may affect through nursing actions.

The scientific processes of research and theory construction are inappropriate for "testing" ideologies. Such processes are useful for developing explanatory knowledge necessary for rationalized nursing actions directed at patient phenomena of concern to practitioners. Confusion as to what nursing theories or models are, or should be, has led to the absurdity of a number of highly abstract orienting models, which have not produced much but general orientations while many nurse researchers engage in disparate, often fragmented, atheoretical research that is not related to, nor reflective of, a clearly articulated nursing framework. As a consequence, one cannot point to any cohesive growing body of nursing practice knowledge. Not much scientific knowledge for nursing practice has been produced by nursing research.

There is heightened awareness of how nurses think as nurses. As Johnson (1974) has stated, "a profession's service to society is an intellectual one" (p. 372). Responsible nurses must examine and reexamine how we acquire and represent knowledge; they must constantly question the state and adequacy of knowledge for professional practice. The societal value of nursing and nurses' contribution to people's health depends upon that adequacy.

Recognition of the continuities and commonalities in the various conceptual models of nursing, as well as the differences, has been rewarding. There is little argument as to the modalities or strategies that characterize nursing as a practice. Compensating, supporting, monitoring, or assessing health states or health behaviors, educating, and consulting are generally accepted modalities for nurses. More controversial and less clear is whether nursing includes distinctive therapies and whether nurses should be problem centered or health and person centered. Nurses have usually claimed to care for persons not diseases, yet focus on problems per se, or taxonomies of problem states, have the potential to weaken a centering on the person rather than on a diagnosis.

The evolution of conceptual models and attention to theoretical thinking of nurses has shown there is agreement that client or patient being and well being are to be maintained or enhanced, and that meaning in nursing comes from the meanings and linkages of the terms *person, client,* or *patient,* with those of *nursing, health,* and *environment.* Nurses agree on these words as essential in any discussion of nursing. They do not agree upon the exact meaning for each term and how *persons* and *environment* are to be linked vis-à-vis the focus and strategies for actions of the nurses. It is agreed that nursing has to do with client, person, or patient responses and behaviors, thoughts and feelings, physical and mental states, and health. Nursing has to do with how people act, react, or behave in the interests of their health. With these several agreements, to some extent the answer to "What is nursing?" has emerged from nursing scholarship.

The answer is dynamic because it must constantly be updated, examined, clarified, and questioned. The goal intended from nursing practice is beneficence. Current conceptual models present nursing as goal-oriented. The models do vary in the specification of the particular beneficence, e.g., self-care competence, adaptation, health, but beneficence for others called patients or clients is clearly the raison d'etre, the justification, and the source of social value, for nursing practice. Nursing practice is the only justification for nursing education or nursing research.

Heightened awareness among nurses of how nurses think as nurses, and attempts to create cohesive *systems* of concepts (Kim, 1983) has begun. Increasingly nurses are engaging in concept analysis and concept clarification. Such activity, vitally needed, is beginning to indicate how nursing meanings depend upon relationships among concepts. Nurses are not as yet effectively producing a system or body of knowledge that enhances or advances nursing practice or that expedites the education and socialization of generations of competent practitioners or investigators. Failure in this respect is due to the failure to attend to the structure of nursing as a field of inquiry. Donaldson and Crowley (1977) suggested approaches to structuring nursing practice knowledge. They began examination of nursing as a field of inquiry, and sketched out themes to identify the domain of nursing as a field of inquiry. Little has been done to critique or advance the conception begun by Donaldson and Crowley.

Concern for nursing research and nursing theory development led to mistakes generally detrimental for organizing knowledge or for structuring knowledge development in the context of a discipline with domain, specified phenomena, significant questions for research, and explicated conceptual and syntactical structures. One major mistake was to argue processes and terms to the neglect of systematic delineation of phenomena of paramount importance to the discipline of nursing. Failure to distinguish, yet relate, nursing as a practice and nursing as a field of inquiry perpetuated a view of nursing as applied science.

Nursing practice obviously, in part, involves the use of generalizations from various sciences. One such generalization is the one which recognizes that humans need oxygenation to survive. The explanations provided by various sciences are used as part of the understandings of human responses and characteristics that nurses in practice must have. Nursing as a field of inquiry, however, is not solely concerned with the applicability of theories from other fields of inquiry though applicability may need to be studied. Nursing as a field of inquiry must also be concerned with development and organization of knowledge about health behaviors, health assets, and health states from a perspective that reflects the nature and conceptualization of nursing practice. In this endeavor nursing as a field of inquiry is distinctive, and is basic to nursing practice. It is inquiry about phenomena not necessarily conceived by, or of interest to other investigators. It is inquiry to produce knowledge for nursing practice not now being produced by other perspectives or by the subject matters of other disciplines.

Selected patient phenomena are what nurses as practitioners attempt to change for the better, maintain, or perhaps fix. They are observable as patient or client states or behaviors that are susceptible to scientific description and explanation. They are states, behaviors, or responses that nurses in practice can observe.

They are observables, as distinguished from concepts or meanings. Treating concepts in isolation, reification, and failure to recognize that concepts are ideas or meanings that require ties to empirical experience, or to some cohesive system of concepts for meanings has led to fragmented ideations with inadequate referents for practical usefulness.

Another mistake, resulting from emphasis on certain research methods, led to inadequate attention to systematic descriptions of nursing phenomena, of what it is that nurses fix, alter, or maintain through nursing modalities. It is all too common for research reports to acknowledge that too little was known about key variables, or the measure of them, for nursing meanings. Clear, observation-based descriptions of the alterable variables that nurses fix, alter, regulate, or maintain through nursing modalities have not been adequately produced. What alterable client or patient variables, under what conditions, may require nursing for stable maintenance? These alterable patient variables are, in part, the subject matter for nursing as a field of inquiry. They have not received sufficient attention from nurse researchers or scholarly practitioners.

While nurses debate methods or stances such as subjectivity versus objectivity, holistic versus particularistic, pragmatism versus idealism, induction versus deduction, empirical versus theoretical, humanistic or naturalistic versus experimental, qualitative versus quantitative, they rarely specify or describe nursing phenomena in detail from skillful, extended observations.

Debates have been relatively sterile. The tendency is to defend rather than explicate or demonstrate. Until subject matter for nursing as a field of inquiry is specified as a field of phenomena not abstract concepts, issues of methods or approaches are inconsequential. Significant questions about important nursing practice phenomena must determine specific research methods. Endless debates on methods, models, and definitions has slowed the development of a community of scholars concerned with development or organization of knowledge useful for improvement of nursing practice.

Current conceptual models may serve some purpose as general orientations, but such general, high-level abstractions do not directly specify the research questions and phenomena to be understood in the discrete and diverse arenas of specialty practices that exist in contemporary nursing practice. Until the questions and phenomena are specified more concretely, nursing research cannot make the contribution to the advancement of practice that it should.

Theories that provide understanding of patient responses, of variability in patterns of behaviors, not grand general conceptualizations of nursing or of man, environment, or health, are needed to advance practice.

Some lines of research in nursing have addressed patient responses in the context of nursing practice, and have contributed to improvement of practice. They have increased practitioners' understanding. They have begun to provide the recognition of the many variables that might need to be considered by practitioners in the design or selection of intervention, or systems for care, for particular persons, situations, and conditions. Theory development about pain management begun by Jacox (1977), or that by Johnson et al. (1970, 1978) on alternative approaches to prepare patients for noxious or potentially aversive stimuli, are examples of scholarship that has been useful to practice and provoked better questions and further research to improve the ability of practitioners to discriminate and select interventions. The work of Schwartz, Henley, and Leitz (1964) on the needs of the elderly ambulatory patient is a hallmark in gerontological research.

Concerted efforts of practitioners and researchers to delineate nursing as a field of inquiry distinct from, but concerned with nursing as a practice is needed. Nursing as a practice is sometimes so affected by situational particulars that activities of nurses and those of other practitioners may overlap somewhat. Nursing as a field of inquiry is distinct by reason of perspective, phenomena, questions, and purposes. Nursing often has failed to distinguish the many meanings of the word *nursing;* profession, activities of nurses, a clinical practice, a field in education, and a field of inquiry. The focus, processes, and goals of these different meanings of *nursing* are different. Failure to appreciate the differences has vitiated nursing as a field of inquiry. It should be recognized, however, that nurses have not been involved in research for very long and that relatively few nurses have been engaged in research. Perhaps impatience and unrealistic expectations of nursing researchers are symptoms of naiveté about the time required for knowledge development in nursing.

REFERENCES

Abdellah, F. G. (1970). Overview of nursing research 1955–1968. *Nursing Research, 19,* 6–17, 151–162, 239–252.

Austin, A. L. (1957). *History of nursing source book.* New York: Putnam's.

Beckstrand, J. (1980). A critique of several conceptions of practice theory in nursing. *Research in Nursing and Health, 3,* 69–79.

Beckstrand, J. (1984). A reply to Collins and Fielder: The concept of theory. *Research in Nursing and Health, 7,* 189–196.

Bridgeman, M. (1953). *Collegiate education for nursing.* New York: Russell Sage Foundation.

Brown, A. F. (1953). *Research in nursing.* Philadelphia: Saunders.

Collins, R. J., & Fielder, J. H. (1981). Beckstrand's concept of practice theory: A critique. *Research in Nursing and Health, 4,* 317–321.

Dickhoff, J., James, P., & Wiedenbach, E. (1968). Theory in a practice discipline. *Nursing Research, 17,* 415–435, 545–554.

Donaldson, S. K., & Crowley, D. M. (1977). Discipline of nursing: Structure and relationship to practice. *Communicating Nursing Research, 10,* 1–22.

Gortner, S. R. (1980). Nursing research: Out of the past and into the future. *Nursing Research, 29,* 204–207.

Gortner, S. R., & Nahm, H. (1977). An overview of nursing research in the United   States. *Nursing Research, 26,* 10–33.

Jacox, A. K. (Ed.). (1977). *Pain: A source book for nurses and other health professionals.* Boston: Little, Brown and Co.

Johnson, D. E. (1974). Development of theory: A requisite for nursing as a primary health professors. *Nursing Research, 23,* 372–377.

Johnson, J. E., Dobbs, J. M., Jr., & Leventhal, H. (1970). Psychological factors in   the welfare of surgical patients. *Nursing Research, 19,* 18–29.

Johnson, J. E., Fuller, S. S., Endress, M. P., & Rice, V. H. (1978). Altering patient responses to surgery: An extension and replication. *Research in Nursing and Health, 1,* 111–121.

Kim, H. S. (1983). *The nature of theoretical thinking in nursing.* Norwalk, CN: Appleton-Century-Crofts.

Munhall, P. L. (1982). Nursing philosophy and nursing research: In apposition or opposition? *Nursing Research, 31,* 176–181.

National League for Nursing Education, The Committee on Education (1917). *Standard curriculum for schools of nursing.* New York: Paulus-Ullman.

Orem, D. E. (Ed.). (1979). *Concept formalization in nursing: Process and product.* Boston: Little, Brown and Co.

Schwartz, D., Henley, B., & Leitz, L. (1964). *The elderly ambulatory patient: Nursing and psychological needs.* New York: Macmillan.

Silva, M. C., & Rothbart, D. (1984). An analysis of changing trends in philosophies of science on nursing theory development and testing. *Advances in Nursing Science, 6*(2), 1–13.

Wald, F. S., & Leonard, R. C. (1964). Towards development of nursing practice theory. *Nursing Research, 13,* 309–313.

11

Nursing Research: Diversity in Scientific Inquiry

EDITORS' INTRODUCTION

In the mid-1980s, the debates about the nature of knowledge devel-opment including theory and research in nursing were many. Ellis consistently argued for acceptance of diversity in knowledge devel-opment and research.

The title assigned me, "Diversity in Scientific Inquiry," stimulated some questions, some reflections, and a heartening sense of exciting developments in nursing research. First let me share two of the ques-tions the title raises and briefly comment on the first question before devoting the majority of my time to the second.

My first question was: Why be concerned only with *scientific* in-quiry when discussing nursing research? The second question was: Diversity of *what in* scientific inquiry?

The first question was provoked by my observation that there is a tendency among nurses to think only science if the word "research" is used. Research and science are synonymous only in the literal mean-

Unpublished paper, "Nursing Research: Diversity in Scientific Inquiry" written March 7, 1985.

ing of *re*-search. If one really means *re*-search or search again, then the search process is engaged in order to search *again* for another, hopefully better, explanation for something than the one that exists. Re-searching implies one has a goal of reformulating one's theoretical thinking or one's theory or formalized explanation of something. Theory, theorizing, and searching for better answers, which usually turn out to better questions for further searching, is the dynamic nature of scientific inquiry. But scientific inquiry isn't the only type of inquiry possible and science isn't the only type of knowledge needed by nurses. Our tendency to think only science if we think about inquiry is due, probably, more to history than anything else.

Florence Nightingale's 1860 curriculum included anatomy, physiology, and chemistry. She also wrote that nursing was best learned in an institution in which there was medical research. She wanted nurses to know *whys*, not simply *hows* for the doings of nurses. Since Nightingale's time, nurses have been influenced in their thinking, their educational experiences, and their practice by developments in the sciences that have produced medical knowledge. When nurses have sought to become able to systematically study something they sought the expertise of scientists in our quest for more or better knowledge for nursing practice.

But let's think about knowledge, nursing practice, and nursing research. Nursing research is conducted for purposes of developing and evaluating nursing knowledge. The goal of research is knowledge. Knowledge is not the goal of nursing practice. Beneficence is. Nursing practice does require the *use* of knowledge. It requires the use of general knowledge, the use of nursing knowledge, the use of skills, and the use of self in the context of ethics and nursing values toward a goal of beneficence or good for clients. Though the various conceptual models of nursing differ in exactly how the goal of practice is specified, the meanings of all of the goals can note health in some form and all are *intended* as beneficence.

To actually produce beneficence entails many types of knowledge: moral, social, personal, and scientific at the very least. It also requires knowledge of particulars, of particular persons, or particular settings or situations, or of particular beliefs or cultures. But it is not the knowledge per se that produces beneficence. Beneficence can only come with artful, ethical use of knowledge. There is much more than scientific knowledge that nurses concerned with knowledge development or research need to consider.

Perhaps you can see why the title given me for today causes me first to say: Why only scientific inquiry? I think we need inquiry of at least two additional types: historical inquiry and philosophic inquiry. For me the term "nursing research" includes scientific inquiry, historical inquiry, philosophic inquiry, and something I can label only crudely as nursing technology development.

Scientific inquiry gives us knowledge in the form of laws, theories, or sets of statements that are our explanations of the nature of things. Science organizes and gives meaning to facts in the form of useful generalizations.

Historical inquiry is of a different sort. It has as its goal the explication of comprehensive understandings of events, eras, traditions, institutions or statuses. Some history of nursing as social institution, profession, practice, or occupation can be produced by historians who are not nurses. However, there are many events, ideas, and developments that nurses need to know about to understand the nature of nursing and why we are where we are, and why we think as we think, that may not be of interest to historians in general. There are also some matters for which nursing meanings may require the way of looking at things and deriving meanings that come from being a nurse. Certainly any history of ideas or concept meanings in nursing requires familiarity with the jargon of nursing that nurses acquire. The integration, understanding, and cohesion that historical inquiry can provide is an essential type of inquiry.

A third type of knowledge nurses must have that requires inquiry is that from philosophic inquiry. Philosophic inquiry produces knowledge that is comprehensive and integrative. It is knowledge not of fact, or of meanings from the discovery, organization, or interpretations of *facts*, which is what scientific inquiry produces. Knowledge produced by philosophers is of norms such as ethics, and of roots or foundations of values and ethics. It may be the explication and justification of methods and goals. We need nurses who are philosophers to study ethics or moral norms and their roots and consequences. We need nurses who are philosophers to explicate and clarify the values inherent in the lasting existence and justification of nursing as a social institution. We need nurses who can explicate and clarify the nature of theoretical thinking and conceptual structures in nursing practice and nursing inquiry. Scientist nurses need to know the roots of their approaches to inquiry and also the history of science in nursing. Philosophic inquiry and knowledge from historians can contribute to the maturation of nursing as a field of inquiry and to development of truly professional practitioners who know, value, and build upon their heritage and noble traditions. The organization and development of knowledge cannot be successful without cognizance of purposes, methods, and contributions to understanding nursing provided by the approaches of science, history, and philosophy.

Studies of nursing technologies are also needed. By nursing technologies I mean the techniques required for effective nursing practice. These include therapeutic interpersonal techniques essential to achieve nursing goals, the improvement or development of nursing procedures or apparatuses for nursing care, or of effective educative techniques for use with patients or clients. My list would also include organizational techniques, such as staffing patterns, or organizational innovations to effectively distribute, organize, or create systems of nursing care of services. Evaluation of the effectiveness of all of the various techniques and nursing technology generally, is a responsibility of scholarly professional nurses. Nurse investigators must be involved in the development of nursing science and nursing technology. They must evaluate that science and technology in the context and actuality of nursing practice at some point. We also need to know a great deal more of the nature of artistry in nursing practice.

Now let me turn to my second major question, which was: Diversity of *what* in scientific inquiry? As I reflected on the question the assigned title raised for me, I decided that we have, and ought to have, diversity in scientific inquiry in the following areas:

1. Research questions or problems;
2. The phenomena, objects or subject matters that need to be studied;
3. The methods, approaches, or the syntaxes that are called for in nursing science inquiry; and
4. The goals of inquiry.

Let me now consider what diversity there is in inquiry in each of these four areas and also argue for the need for or value of such diversity.

There is, and ought to be, diversity in the kinds of questions posed by various nurse investigators. Research or inquiry has to do with knowledge development. As nurses came to appreciate research and, of necessity, began to prepare themselves to do research, they focused upon learning how to do it. Early texts on nursing research described *the* scientific method as if there is only one method or way to do scientific inquiry. Some equated research and problem solving not unlike the steps in the problem solving process long advocated as the right approach to use for nursing practice. Nurse educators sought to teach the problem solving process and wrote about it neatly delineating the sequential steps in the process. As we struggled to answer the question "what is nursing?," which cannot be ignored, we came up with the nursing process. And again we delineated, described, and learned the steps in the how to do it. All the apparent fascination or emphasis on processes, on teaching how-to-do-its, may very well explain why in our naivete as to research we have erred in being overly preoccupied with learning, teaching, and arguing methods for nursing research to the neglect of consideration of what to research and the whys of nursing research.

Many undergraduate or masters program courses on research have taught the steps in the research process or how to do it with insufficient delineation of the important knowledge questions to be addressed by whatever methods or ingenuity that may be required by reason of the nature of the questions or phenomena to be studied. It is common in such first research courses to focus only on the testing or validation or justification processes of inquiry. Exercises in formulating and testing hypotheses or testable research questions have their value. First studies, however, often end with the conclusion that not enough was known about the focal variables in the conception and design of the study, and what was learned from doing the study was how little we know about nursing variables. The paucity of adequate descriptions of the phenomena of interest to nurses becomes apparent if one notices how often experimental design studies end up commenting on the inadequate conceptualization or measurement of the variables of importance. So one type of question we need to use, and welcome as a guide to inquiry, would be what is the nature of some-thing?

Before expecting adequate or meaningful hypothesis formulations and testings we need to encourage and support immersion in situations where a phenomenon of interest might be expected to occur. We need to encourage studies that ask questions that produce careful descriptions of the phenomena or of situations or variables associated with the phenomenon. We need studies that clarify our concepts by questions that tie them to phenomena or observables in some reliable and meaningful-for-nursing manner. Descriptive or hypothesis generating studies are not adequately valued in nursing, yet they are sorely needed. Perhaps we have overvalued hypothesis testing or prematurely tried for rigor in validation processes before we really know the nature of our variables.

We have little nursing knowledge as to the processes of discovery, which are as important in understanding what scientific inquiry is as the steps in some problem solving or validation process that has been objectified and numbered or sequenced.

Our neglect of discovery is understandable. Discovery as a process is not reducible to an ordered set of procedures to be followed, or some algorithm. It cannot be taught. It is individualistic; it can be serendipitous. It is a function of mind-set, interest, opportunity, personality, happenstance, and creativity. The processes are uneven and idiosyncratic but are the beginnings of a long process of formulation and familiarization and scrutiny that must precede formal or objectified formulations then controlled testings, reformulation if necessary, then retesting, usually in a cyclical manner.

Total development from wonder to insight to testable question to scientific knowledge moves from the wonder of one individual mind to increasingly impersonal, public, objectifiable, systematized, validated knowledge of a distinctive type called science.

We must foster and support questions of wonder and of exploration and description. Preoccupation with formal methods and design rigor seems to occur in nursing at the expense of discourse on the nature of the important questions to be addressed in a nursing knowledge system. Dominant nursing models vary, but all include humans as a critical element along with other highly abstract complexities. To produce science from such abstractions and data perceivable through some direct or indirect observations must be recognized and overcome in some way.

If one accepts that nursing research requires the concept *humans,* then perforce one must consider what questions about humans must be studied to produce the essential knowledge of humans we think we need in a nursing knowledge system. What human phenomena do we need data on to build the scientific portion of that knowledge system?

Diversity in *questions* is one essential diversity in scientific inquiry in nursing. Questions of wonder are needed. So also are questions that can only be formed from extensive immersion in or contacts with phenomena when such immersion can be done without the blinding constraints of a priori definitions or fixed sets. Such immersions are an essential experience for *hypothesis-generating* questions, which we need in nursing.

There are those who want scientists to have no concern for whether the knowledge they seek is useful. For me, this raises a philosophic question to be studied in nursing. It seems to me we need nursing knowledge not just for the sake of knowing, but the long range sake of doing something. That something is nursing practice that is ethical, humane, efficient, and available.

Diversity in questions is paralleled by diversity in the subject matter or phenomena to be studied. In 1966, the first of a series of four symposia for nursing science development was held at Case Western Reserve. The question posed for that conference was "Research, how will nursing define it?" At the end of the day of papers and discussions by nurses and other scientists, Rozella Schlotfeldt summed up the sense of the discussions by saying it appeared that the question "What is nursing research?" was an improper one. That wasn't Schlotfeldt's personal view; it was her reading of the consensus that day.

In 1932 the Association of Collegiate Schools of Nursing stated one of their goals as support of nursing research. It has taken us over fifty years to come to attempts to articulate the phenomena that are focal for nursing research.

My own past attempts to study the history of nursing research led me to identify that history by periods which are very similar to those Meleis (1985) identifies for the history of theoretical nursing. Those periods that are germane to this presentation are:

1. A period of focus on practice procedures and technique. (Petry study of preparation of hypo).
2. A period of focus on nurses and students of nursing in terms of education and administration.
3. A period of focus on activities and functions of nurses. (Time sampling.)
4. The nurse scientist period and focus on research methods, tools, and concepts often shaped by influence of behavioral or natural sciences.
5. The present, which reflects all of the above, but has finally begun to include focus on patient or client states, behaviors or responses, or other phenomena that is clinical.

I recently looked back at the report of the 1967 Nursing Science Symposium at Case Western Reserve. It was on theory development in nursing. The questions the speakers had been asked to address was "What theory is needed?" What kind, and about what? Specifically they were to consider whether nurses should be concerned with general theories of humans, with theories about nurses or patients as special subsets of humans, with theories of nurse–client interactions, or with theories about patients.

Eighteen years later we have the same unanswered questions and haven't produced any cohesive body of nursing science knowledge. More nurses now are thinking about theory development and nursing research and we are now saying *human responses* instead of patient responses, but that is not a great deal of progress in eighteen years. One explanation for our slowness is perhaps the ambiguities and confusion arising from multiple meanings of abstract terms such as model, meta-paradigm, conceptual framework, and the like. When the confusion is compounded by relative naivete about the nature of science and what we intend to mean by the term *nursing* science, we dissipate our efforts in talking about research and about theory instead of about nursing questions or nursing phenomena, or instead of doing nursing research or further developing nursing theories about nursing phenomena of all sorts.

A third area in which we have some diversity, but have begun lately to debate rather fruitlessly is that of method or the syntax of our discipline. Why *debate?* Or *discuss?* Maybe I could be led to believe that at least dialectic discourse might have value. But I think that any form of verbal argument on methods is premature until we specify the nature of the significant questions of the discipline and the phenomena to be explained, understood, controlled, or predicted. These phenomena must include those empirical realities that nurses as practitioners manipulate, or change in the cause of beneficence, or seek to preserve or maintain for the comatose trauma victim, the vulnerable elderly person, or the premature infant, for example. Because these nursing practice phenomena are out there observable empirical realities does not, however, mean that nursing science is produced or to be produced only by the empirical method.

I find debates pitting empirical vs. theoretical, qualitative vs. quantitative, objectivity vs. subjectivity, experimental vs. naturalistic, and such rather pointless. They represent our adulation and focus on process instead of on questions and phenomena. It is the significance and nature of the nursing research questions and phenomena that must determine the appropriate methods for inquiry. We can learn from many sources and experiences. We need to be open to diversity in methods. We may need to create methods that are those dictated by our questions and our phenomena, our goals and our perspective.

There are four approaches or "habits of thinking" (Zbilut, 1978, p. 128) that have been viewed as useful for studying human nature. All have been used to seek nursing knowledge. The four are:

1. emperiological–experiential (scientific research and personal experience);
2. empirical–metaphenomenal (hypothesis, theory, law);
3. philosophical–metaphenomenal (human contingencies of man's existence); and
4. philosophical–transcendental.

All of these approaches to understanding humans offer something for nursing inquiry, but approach can only be considered if one knows the question one has asked about the phenomenon to be studied. Methods depend upon the question and cannot be considered with any meaning apart from questions, or the nature of the perplexities we seek to extinguish, the knowledge problems we cannot ignore. We must learn to judge investigations by the significance of the question researched and by the value or usefulness of the research product for a nursing knowledge system or for nursing practice.

A final topic I feel I must address, though diversity is not a necessary concept or essential consideration for the topic, is that of pure or basic science versus applied or clinical science. I question the necessity of making the distinction. The distinction *is* made however by those who call nursing or nursing science an applied science.

Mulkay (1977) distinguished pure or basic science and applied science in terms of the social context in which research is undertaken. Pure research is intended for, and communicated to other scientists. The criteria for its evaluation are scientific. Applied research by contrast, is undertaken on behalf of "laymen" and is communicated to laymen for their use for purposes other than the further extension of scientific knowledge. In the nursing community can we afford to imagine our colleagues in practice as our "laymen" if we are scientist nurses? Or should we value our common dominant identity as nurses?

Leininger in 1969 wrote that the "goal of any scientific field is to accurately describe phenomena, to explain and compare different orders of phenomena, and to ultimately predict and control phenomena under investigation" (p. 484). Who are members of the scientific field called nursing?

Leininger also wrote:

> It is generally recognized that nursing is primarily an applied field because the professional members draw heavily upon knowledge from the natural sciences, social sciences, and the humanities. Will nursing remain as an applied science in the future? If not, what factors need to be considered to make it a pure science? Should nursing endeavor to be both an applied and a pure science? (p. 484)

How realistic or useful is it to say the pure scientist is working for the sake of knowledge per se while the applied scientist is primarily involved in the use of knowledge produced by the pure scientist? Leininger noted in 1969 that a third view had emerged. It is that it is an impossible and a futile argument to maintain a sharp distinction between a pure and an applied scientific field. The integrator view considers knowledge from pure science inherently implies application to practical life problems. For nursing as a knowledge field the artificial dichotomy makes no sense within nursing. Further, it makes no sense for nursing as a discipline if we no longer define nursing science as only that derived from other sciences and transformed for use in nursing practice. (If we still use that old definition of nursing science then there is no nursing research or need for it.)

Kaplan (1964) writes:

> The fact is that the distinction between "pure" and "applied" science, whatever its logical ground is not of much help in understanding the actual growth of knowledge. (p. 398)

> An inquiry which is specifically directed at the solution of some practical problem is not for that reason alone to be excluded from the category of basic research. (p. 199)

Nursing practice is the ultimate raison d'etre of all else in nursing. Ideally every nurse needs to be simultaneously expert practitioner, brilliant creative scientist, great humanitarian, noble statesperson, and dedicated scholar. Lacking realization of this impossible dream, we need each other. We must be a community of nurses and use our various diversities for their strengths and contributions.

REFERENCES

Kaplan, A. (1964). *The conduct of inquiry: Methodology for behavioral science.* San Francisco: Chandler Publishing Co.

Leininger, M. (1969). Ethnoscience: A New and Promising Research Approach for the Health Sciences, *Image, 3*(1), 2–8.

Meleis, A. I. (1985). *Theoretical nursing: Development & progress.* Philadelphia: J.B. Lippincott.

Mulkay, M. J. (1977). Sociology of the scientific research community. In I. Spiegel-Rösing & D. J. de Solla Price (Eds.), *Science, technology and society* (pp. 93–148). London: Sage.

Zbilut, J. P. (1978). Epistemologic constraints to the development of a theory of nursing (Letter to the Editor). *Nursing Research 27*(2), 128–129.

Index